LIVING WITH DISABILITY

DETAILS OF AUTHORS

Gillian Johnson obtained her first degree at the University of Oxford and her diplomas in social work from the University of Glasgow. She has worked in a local authority social work department and carried out this project with her husband, as a research worker in the University departments of Neurology and Social Administration, Glasgow.

Ralph Johnson studied Medicine at the University of Cambridge and University College Hospital and was later Lecturer in Neurology at the University of Oxford and Dean of St Peters College in that University. This project was carried out while he was Senior Lecturer in Neurology in the University of Glasgow and Consultant Neurologist at the Institute of Neurological Sciences in Glasgow. He is now Dean and Professor of Medicine of the University of Otago responsible for the Clinical School of Medicine, Wellington, New Zealand.

Living with

A SURVEY OF SOCIAL SERVICES SUPPORT FOR MULTIPLE SCLEROSIS PATIENTS IN SCOTLAND

GILLIAN and RALPH JOHNSON

CHURCHILL LIVINGSTONE
Medical Division of Longman Group Limited

Distributed in the United States of America by Longman Inc., 19 West 44th Street, New York, N.Y. 10036 and by associated companies, branches and representatives throughout the world.

First Published 1978

ISBN 0 443 01696 8

British Library Cataloging in Publication Data
Johnson, Gillian S
Living with disability.
1. Social work with the physically handicapped – Scotland – Glasgow 2. Multiple sclerosis – Scotland – Glasgow
I. Title II. Johnson, Ralph Hudson
362.4'3'0941443 HV3024.G7 78–40009

Printed in Great Britain by
Lowe & Brydone Printers Limited, Thetford, Norfolk

Preface

This report gives the results of a survey carried out among 104 patients with multiple sclerosis in the Glasgow Region. The aim of the project was to examine the problems they encountered living in the community, and the availability of employment and social services to them. As a result of the findings we recommend reorganisation of the services by the establishment of regular clinics at which the patients would be registered.

We are grateful to all the MS patients who took part in the survey. We also thank Dr. F. Williams and the University of Glasgow Computing Service for assistance in processing data, the neurological consultants, Institute of Neurological Sciences, Glasgow, for letting us contact their patients and Mrs J. Lodge for typing the Report. The work was supported by Grants from the Scottish Branch of the Multiple Sclerosis Society and from IBM (UK) Ltd. A grant towards publication is gratefully acknowledged from Dr. I.D. Melville's Research Fund. Table 1 and Figure 1 are reproduced by kind permission of Professor J.N. Walton and the Oxford University Press.

In this account the following abbreviations are used:

MS	Multiple Sclerosis
MS Society	Multiple Sclerosis Society
INS	Institute of Neurological Sciences Southern General Hospital, Glasgow
DRO	Disablement Resettlement Officer
MSW	Medical Social Worker
LASW	Local Authority Social Worker

Summary

A survey has been carried out of 104 patients with multiple sclerosis (MS) in the West of Scotland. All patients were living at home and we examined the success of services to assist them in the community. The patients were aged 16 to 65 years and had permanent disability, many being severely handicapped. Regular hospital follow-up was more common among the least disabled. Twenty-four patients had never seen a social worker. Many patients had experienced problems with employment but 37 per cent of these had never registered with a Disablement Resettlement Officer. After advice 10 additional patients applied successfully for an attendance allowance. Legislation requires local authorities to compile a register of the disabled and give information on services available to them. Only 19 however were registered and no one had received any information from a local authority. We conclude that many of these MS sufferers had failed to establish or maintain contact with available services. We suggest that these results indicate a need for reorganisation of the support for the chronically disabled, possibly by setting up regular clinics for assessment and management as recommended by the 'Tunbridge' Report (1972).

The results have been briefly reported in an article in the *Lancet* (Johnson and Johnson, 1977).

Contents

Details of multiple sclerosis

Multiple Sclerosis (MS) is a disease of the central nervous system (the brain and spinal cord). The clinical findings are described in standard neurological texts such as Walton (1977) and recent review articles include those of Johnson and McLellan (1972) and McAlpine (1973). Sources for references and summaries of most aspects of the disease include the monograph by McAlpine, Lumsden and Acheson (1972) and the report 'Multiple Sclerosis' from the Office of Health Economics (1975). The following notes provide background information to aid understanding of the social problems which have been examined in this survey.

Pathology

The disease results from dysfunction of nerve fibres in the central nervous system, the most characteristic feature being damage to the myelin sheath which surrounds nerve fibres, thus interfering with the normal passage of nerve impulses along the fibres. The damage, known as demyelination, tends to occur in scattered patches which extend as the disease progresses. Although the process of demyelination is irreversible some of the symptoms occur because of surrounding oedema (or swelling) which may resolve. Improvement may therefore occur if the oedema disappears. The causation of the demyelination is not understood. Many theories have been advanced, including dietary factors, viral infection and an immunological etiology. The evidence is discussed by the authors mentioned above and by Behan and Johnson (1975) and Davison *et al.*, (1975).

Symptoms

The symptoms of MS vary from one patient to another and at different times within the experience of one patient. They may include paraesthesiae (tingling sensations), numbness, muscle weakness and poor co-ordination, slurred speech, visual disorders and disturbances of thought or mood. The symptoms with which the disease may present have been analysed by Walton (1977) (Table 1). Early symptoms may occur rapidly, in days or even hours, frequently increasing in severity over a period of weeks. However, there may then be a considerable period during which the patient apparently returns to normal and the first symptoms may be forgotten until the disease manifests

Table 1 The first symptoms of multiple sclerosis in a series of 100 consecutive patients with the disease (Walton, 1977 by kind permission)

WEAKNESS OR LOSS OF CONTROL OVER LIMBS	No.
Involving both lower limbs	18
Involving one lower limb	14
Involving one upper limb	9
Involving one upper and one lower limb	7
Involving all four limbs	12
	60
VISUAL SYMPTOMS	
'Blindness' in one eye	16
Double vision	8
'Dimness' of vision	4
Homonymous field defect	1
	29
SENSORY SYMPTOMS	
Numbness and other painless paraesthesiae	11
MISCELLANEOUS SYMPTOMS	
Vertigo	2
Tremor	2
Multiple symptoms	2
Ptosis	1
Loss of taste	1
Epilepsy	1
Impotence	1
	10

itself more severely at a later date. In a few patients it is possible that the disease does not develop. Because of this pattern and the lack of clear diagnostic tests it is often difficult to date the onset of the disease.

The typical pattern of multiple sclerosis consists of recurrent exacerbations and remissions, but there is considerable variability in the way the disease may develop (Fig. 1). During a relapse the patient may be severely disabled and confined to bed or admitted to hospital, but between attacks the condition of the patient may improve to a state similar to that which existed prior to the attack, although there is usually some deterioration. The pattern of symptoms which occurred at an earlier attack tends to return in later relapses, with the addition of new symptoms and signs as the disease progresses.

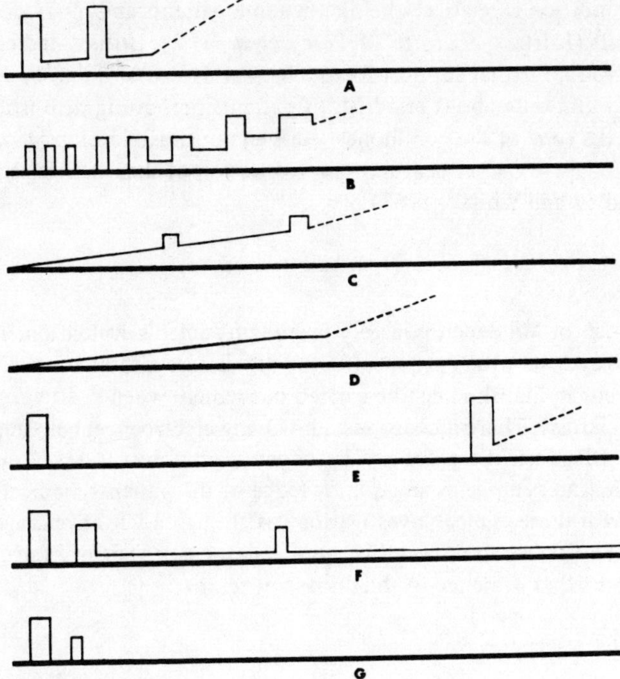

Fig. 1 The course of multiple sclerosis. The line diagrams A – G indicate different modes of development. The vertical blocks indicate exacerbations and increasing slope indicates gradual deterioration. Absence of a continuing line (in E – G) is intended to suggest that the disease is quiescent with no physical signs or symptoms (Brain, 1962, by kind permission).

The intervals between relapses varies from one patient to another and may be weeks, months or years. Some patients experience such long periods of remission that the disease appears to be static. The usual result, however, is a gradual progression of irreversible neurological changes and development of disability. Thus the patient may develop severe problems with co-ordination of upper and lower limbs and become so paralysed that he is unable to walk. Further evidence of severe spinal cord involvement is the frequent development of bladder and bowel incontinence. Mental function is relatively well preserved in many patients but 25% have a reactive depression and nearly two thirds suffer from some degree of mental deterioration; it is in such patients that euphoria is found. In only a small proportion (about 6.5 per cent), however, is there severe intellectual deterioration (Surridge, 1969).

The length of time between onset of symptoms and death is very variable. In a few patients the disease may be so benign that it may not affect life span, whereas some patients may succumb in less than five years. It is now recognised that the condition is relatively benign in some patients and 69-74 per cent live 25 years (Kurtzke *et al.*, 1970; Percy *et al.*, 1971; British Medical Journal, 1972). Further support for the benign nature of the disease was the finding that only about one fifth of patients presenting with isolated optic neuritis (one of the commonest early symptoms) develop MS within ten years; of these 64 per cent have no restriction of their activities at that stage (Bradley and Whitty, 1968).

Diagnosis

The diagnosis of MS depends largely on the physician's evaluation. There are no laboratory tests which are specific for the disease although certain tests on the cerebrospinal fluid can be carried out which, when positive, suggest multiple sclerosis. There are also tests involving electroencephalographic responses. Diagnosis therefore usually depends on observations of neurological signs and symptoms and a knowledge of the patients medical history, together with these clinical investigations. Although a tentative diagnosis may be made at a first examination this can often not be confirmed until a later date when further evidence of the disease develops.

Treatment

Many forms of therapy have been suggested corresponding to the different theories which have been proposed to account for the disease. Unfortunately no treatment has withstood the rigors of scientific testing. Thus although it appears that steroid therapy (especially adrenocorticotrophic hormone, ACTH) has a favourable affect on recent relapses there is no evidence that it influences outcome. Similar observations have been made on the use of a diet containing polyunsaturated fatty acids such as sun-flower seed oil. Details of these approaches to treatment may be found in the references and reviews already quoted. Because of the failure of medical therapy at the present time to ameliorate the disease there is a corresponding need to consider the social and economic problems it creates.

Introduction to the survey

The deficiencies of the social and medical support of patients with chronic disability living in the community were highlighted by the passing of the Chronically Sick and Disabled Persons Act (1970). This gave details of services which should be available to the disabled, and required local authorities to identify the disabled in their area and to provide information of the services available to them. The need for this development in Scotland, which had been excluded from the 1970 Act, was shown by our observations of the shortcomings in the provision of social services for paraplegics in the West of Scotland (Johnson and Johnson, 1972, 1973). This provided evidence which led to the introduction of the Chronically Sick and Disabled Persons (Scotland) Act, (1972). Despite the apparent failure of community support there has been no co-ordinated identification of the disabled and their problems ('The Missing Million' report by the National Fund for Research into Crippling Diseases, 1975).

A detailed examination of the services available to patients with multiple sclerosis (MS) has been carried out and is described here. The results show that the facilities available to these patients are frequently inadequate. Reorganisation of the services for them and for other patients with disabilities should be considered, as suggested in the report on Rehabilitation produced by the committee of the Department of Health and Social Security chaired by Sir Ronald Tunbridge (1972). We recommend that such reorganisation should receive urgent examination and its costs might be less than those of the present patchy and often duplicated services.

Survey methods

Selection of patients

The selection of patients with MS was made from two sources: the MS Society list of patient members in Glasgow and the diagnostic list of the University Department of Neurology at the INS, Glasgow. All patient members of the MS Society knew that they were suffering from MS. The patients from the INS came from Glasgow and surrounding counties as it is the main neurological centre for the West of Scotland; we were aware that they would not always know their diagnosis.

The criteria for selection of patients for study were that they were between the ages of 16 years and 65 years, as such patients would normally be expected to be in employment with financial and social independence, that they should be living at home and have some degree of permanent disability. The final sample of 104 patients with MS who took part in the survey was obtained as follows (Fig. 2):

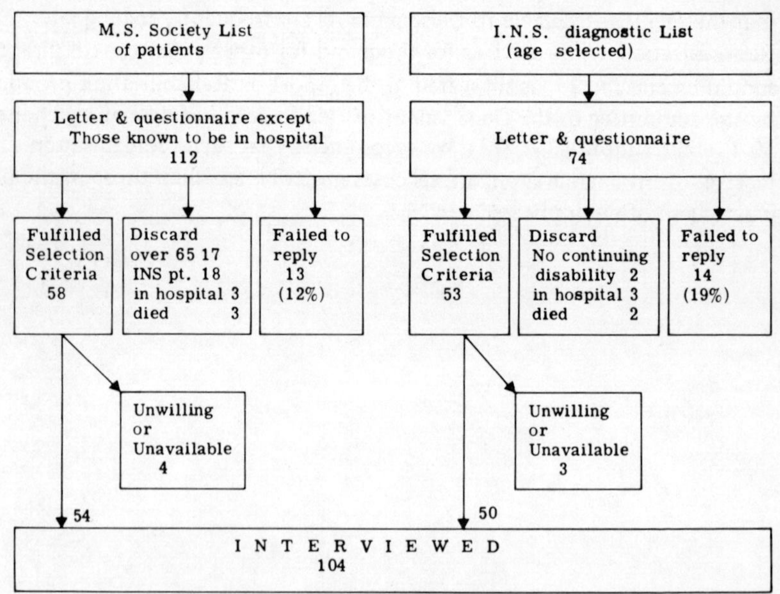

Fig. 2 The method of selection of the 104 patients with MS who were interviewed.

All members of the Glasgow Branch of the MS Society, except for those who were known to be long term patients in hospital, were contacted by letter. Enclosed with the letter was a stamped addressed envelope and a small questionnaire which the recipient was asked to return in order to allow selection on the basis of age and continuing disability. MS Society members who stated that they had attended the INS were excluded. Of 112 people contacted 99 replied. Forty-one of these were unsuitable for inclusion in the survey, 2 declined to participate and at the interviewing stage two other patients were unable to take part. Thus 54 patients were interviewed (76 per cent of the total of those fulfilling criteria for selection plus those who failed to reply). Where possible the respondents were contacted by telephone in order to arrange an interview. Those who did not give a telephone number were sent a second letter suggesting a date and time for an interview, and a stamped postcard was enclosed for return to indicate whether or not the time was suitable. Those members who were not to be included in the survey were sent a letter thanking them for their reply and explaining that their further assistance was not required.

The names of all patients who had attended the University Department of Neurology (INS) during the previous three years and who had been diagnosed as suffering from MS were obtained from the hospital with the consent of the consultants. Patients who had any additional disorder were eliminated from the sample. Further reductions were made according to the selection criteria leaving a potential sample of 74 who were contacted as before. In addition they were asked to state their diagnosis, if known. Sixty patients replied. Seven of these did not fulfil the selection criteria, two were unwilling to take part, and one was unavailable for interview. This left 50 patients who were interviewed (75 per cent of the total of those fulfilling criteria for selection plus those who failed to reply).

As in the group chosen from the MS Society, interviews were arranged by telephone and where this was not possible a letter was sent to each patient enclosing a stamped postcard in order to arrange a suitable time for interview.

Interviews

Two pilot interviews were carried out during the design stage of the questionnaire. All interviews were conducted personally by visiting the patients in their homes. The interview time was usually about two hours. A questionnaire, which was completed during the interview, allowed information to be standardised and computerised. The questionnaire was divided into two parts:

The *first* dealt with physical state. The patients were asked about the extent of their disability under the following headings:

Effect on upper limbs
Effect on lower limbs
Bladder and bowel dysfunction
Speech defect
Visual change
Mental change

The information obtained was subjective, being the patient's personal assessment, together with observations made by the interviewer. Patients were then asked to state what difficulty they had in performing tasks involved in daily living (dressing, brushing hair, etc.), writing and fine precision movements involving the hand and fingers (such as doing up buttons). The effect of the disorder upon walking was indicated by whether or not the individual used a walking aid or wheelchair. The *second* section included questions on social problems. Additional information was also noted.

Interviews were often attended by other members of the family who were free to add comments and give further information. In a few cases, where the patient's speech was badly impaired, the questions were answered with the help of a relative. Only one patient, however, had the questionnaire answered entirely by a relative as she was unable to understand the questions being asked. Interviewing took place between February, 1973 and August, 1974.

Questionnaire to Local Authorities

After the interviews were completed a questionnaire was sent to the four local authority divisions in the survey area (Glasgow, Dunbarton, Lanark, Renfrew) in order to obtain information on the current provision of services and plans for future development.

Results

The results have been briefly reported in an article in the *Lancet* (Johnson and Johnson, 1977).

Details of subjects

Age and sex (Fig. 3)

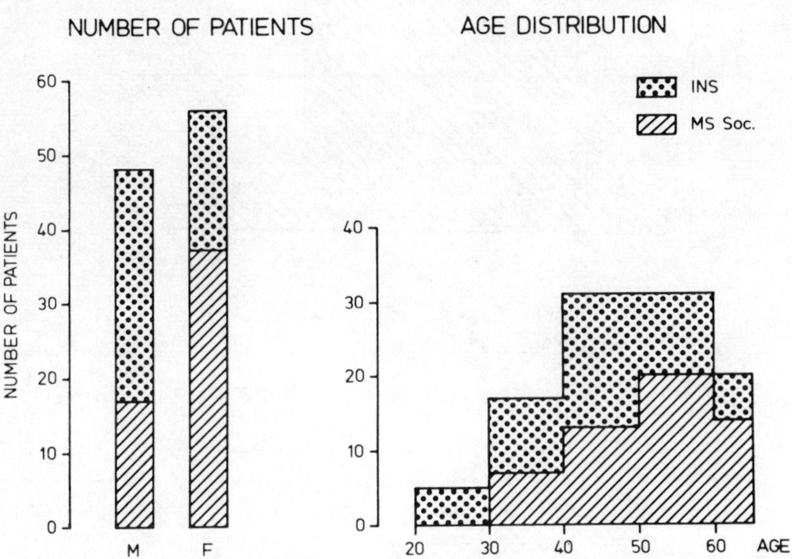

Fig. 3 The age and sex distribution of patients from the INS and MS Society.

Forty-eight males and 56 females were interviewed. In the group drawn from the INS there were 31 males and 19 females while the members of the MS Society consisted of 17 males and 37 females. The age of those interviewed ranged from 20 years to 65 years. Among the INS patients the greatest number occurred in the range 40-50 years. There were more MS Society members between 50-60 years and none of its members was under the age of 30 years.

Age at onset and duration of disability (Figs. 4,5)

The mean age at onset of the disease was 30-40 years but there was a wide distribution. The majority of patients had been disabled for more than 5 years.

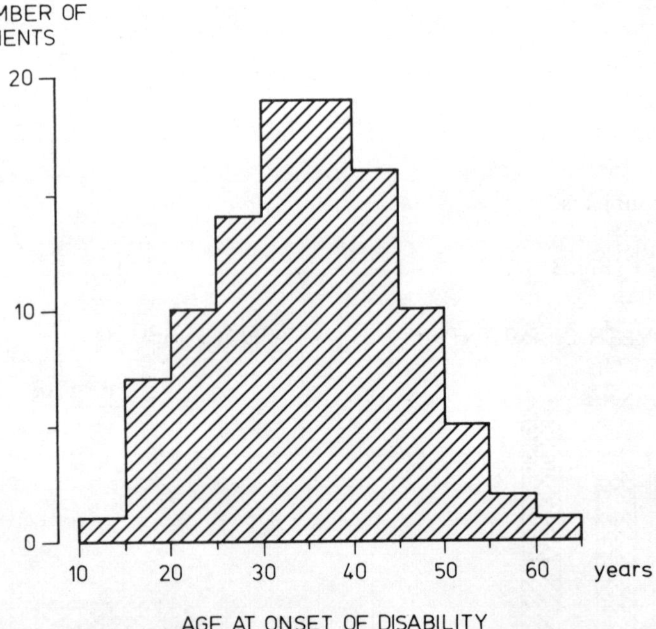

Fig. 4 The age at onset of MS in all patients.

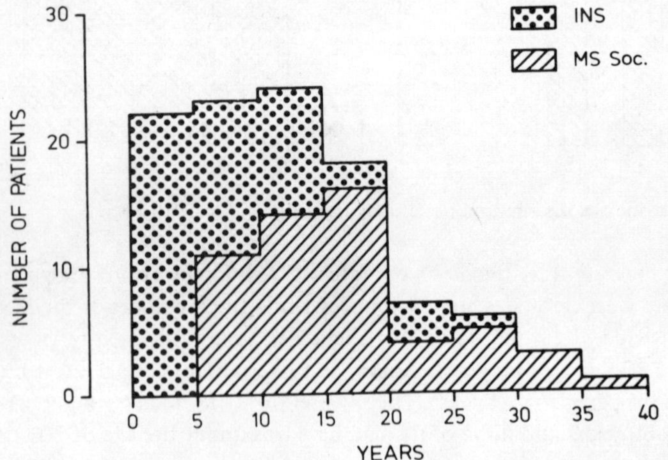

Fig. 5 The duration of disability according to group in INS and MS Society patients.

On average MS Society members had been disabled for longer than patients from the INS.

Marital status (Fig.6)

There were 79 married and 17 single MS patients. Six had got married after the onset of MS. Three others were widowed, one was separated and there were 4 divorcees. Three of the divorces and the separation had occurred after the partner had developed MS but the significance of the disease in the breakdown of the marriages was not examined.

Of those who were married, or had been married, 66 had children. In 17 instances one or more children had been born after one of the partners had developed the first symptoms of MS. Three other couples had adopted children, and in one case a child had been adopted after the adoptive father had developed MS. He had already successfully adopted one child, however, before the onset of disability.

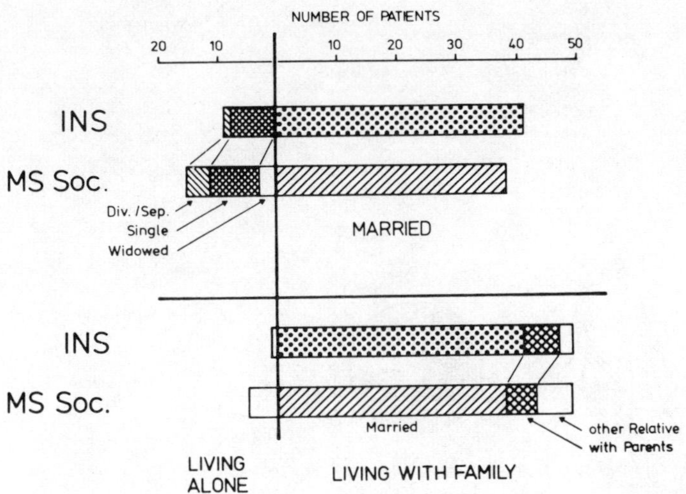

Fig. 6 The marital status of INS and MS Society patients (above). The family support of patients in the two groups (below).

Extent of disability

Upper limbs (Fig. 7a). Ninety-seven patients had motor involvement of the upper limbs, 10 experiencing weakness in the arms only and 87 having impaired use of both arms and hands. Sixty-one people stated that this affected their ability to do basic everyday tasks, in 62 it affected handwriting and in 66 fine precision movements, these categories were not mutually exclusive.

Lower limbs (Fig. 7b). Difficulty with walking was experienced by 99 patients, 29 of whom had one leg affected and 70 of whom had both legs affected. Seventy of the total group relied on an aid for mobility, 44 of them using a wheelchair. A further 7 were so severely disabled that they were largely confined to bed. Only 27 were able to walk without the use of any aid.

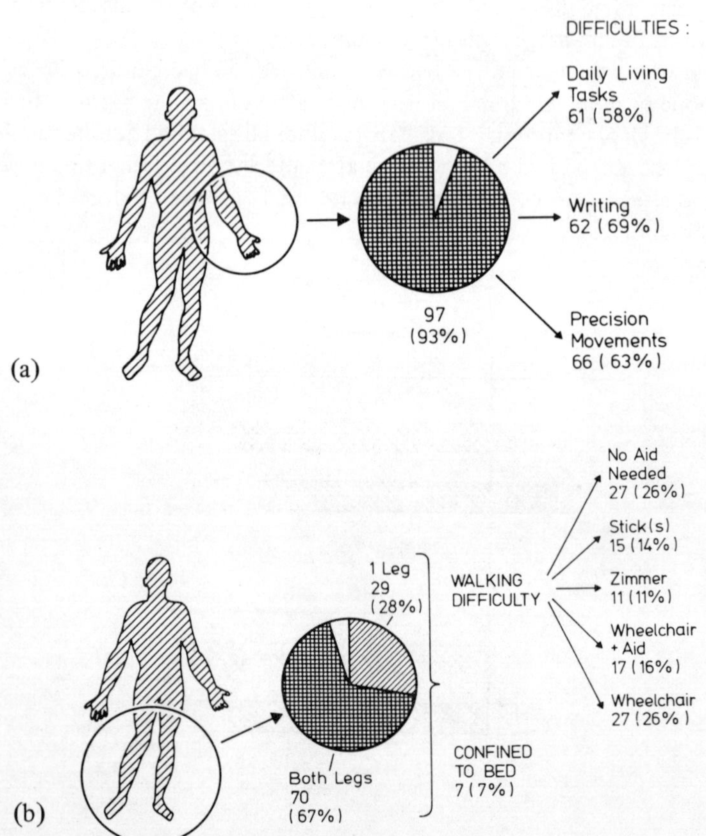

Fig. 7 Motor disabilities experienced by the patients in upper limbs (a, above) and in legs (b, below).

Bladder and/or bowel dysfunction (Fig. 8a) occurred in 79 patients. Seventy-five said that they had a problem with bladder control and 23 with bowel control. Nineteen of these experienced combined dysfunction of both bladder and bowel and 10 suffered from severe double incontinence.

Involvement of speech; eyes, mental change (Fig. 8b) Fifty-three patients reported a problem with their eyesight. In 35 of these patients it was one of

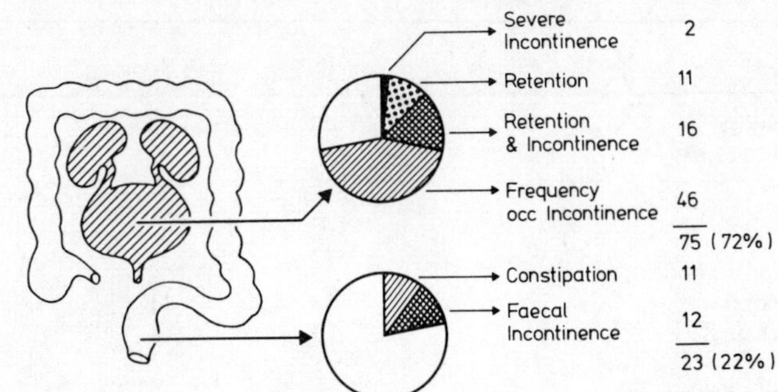

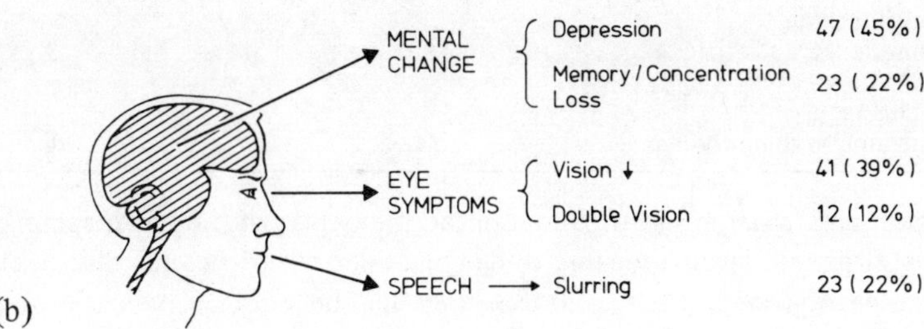

Fig. 8 The frequencies of bladder and bowel dysfunction (a, above) and of mental change, eye symptoms and speech defects (b, below).

general deterioration of sight while 18 experienced episodes of blurred or double vision. Forty-seven patients stated that they experienced phases of depression, 13 that they suffered loss of memory and 10 that they found difficulty in maintaining concentration. These three groups were not mutually exclusive. Some of the information about mental impairment was obtained from relatives.

The breakdown of these groups according to their origins from the INS or the MS Society is given in Table 2. The table indicates that the patients from the MS Society had greater disability than the hospital group.

Knowledge of diagnosis

All the MS Society patients and 43 of the INS patients knew their diagnosis. The seven who did not know that they had MS had been given various names for their disorder by hospital doctors or general practitioners. Their descriptions ranged from neuraesthenia and cervical spondylosis to ‘a serious nervous

Table 2 The disabilities of the two groups of patients
Note: Disability was greater among the MS Society patients

Disabilities	INS	MS Society	Total
Motor disability	43	54	97
arms and hands			
legs			
aids:			
confined to bed	3	4	7)
wheelchair	13	31	44) 74%
zimmer or stick	12	14	26)
Vision deterioration	21	20	41
Bladder dysfunction			
incontinence, frequency, retention	31	44	75
Bowel dysfunction			
incontinence	9	14	23
Mental change			
depression or memory loss	34	36	70

condition' and 'a patch of inflammation on the nerves of the lower spine'. Only two of these seven appeared to be concerned about the diagnosis which they had been given and they said that they 'had been left in the dark'.

As well as those who did not know their diagnosis there were others (7 INS and 3 MS Society patients) who appeared to know little about MS and who said that they had not discussed it with a doctor. In some instances the patient had never been told the diagnosis directly by a doctor but had obtained the information from a relative, or by reading the case notes, or overhearing a discussion among medical staff in a hospital ward. It was common for patients to have consulted a variety of medical books in order to learn more about their disorder.

Employment

Occupation before disability and at time of survey (Fig. 9, Table 3)
Before the onset of diability 76 of the total group were in remunerative employment (Fig. 10). Eighteen of these had professional occupations, 10 clerical, 22 manual skilled and 24 unskilled occupations. Two others were in the armed forces. Of the remaining 28, making up the total group of 104, 25 were housewives, 2 were in full-time education and 1 had retired. No-one was unemployed.

At the time of the survey only 17 were in full-time employment (8 professional, 7 clerical and 2 manual skilled). There were 15 more housewives

Table 3 Occupational category of MS Society and INS patients before disability and at time of interview

	Before disability INS	MS Society	Total	After disability INS	MS Society	Total
Professional	12	6	18	6	2	8
Clerical	3	7	10	7	–	7
Manual skilled	13	9	22	2	–	2
unskilled	6	18	24	–	–	–
H.M. Forces	–	2	2	–	–	–
in remunerative employment	34	42	76	15	2	17
Housewife	13	12	25	15	25	40
Student	1	–	1	–	–	–
School child	1	–	1	–	–	–
Retired	1	–	1	2	–	2
Unemployed	–	–	–	18	27	45
No remunerative employment	16	12	28	35	52	87

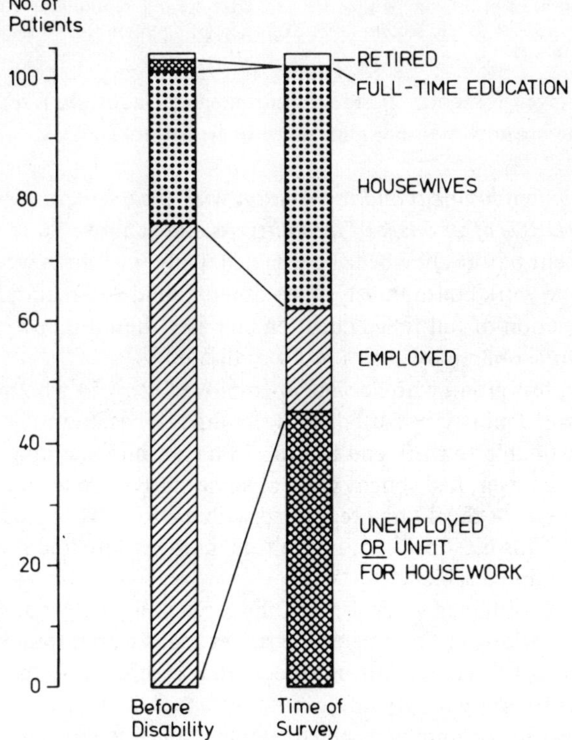

Fig. 9 Occupation of the total group of 104 patients before disability and at the time of survey.

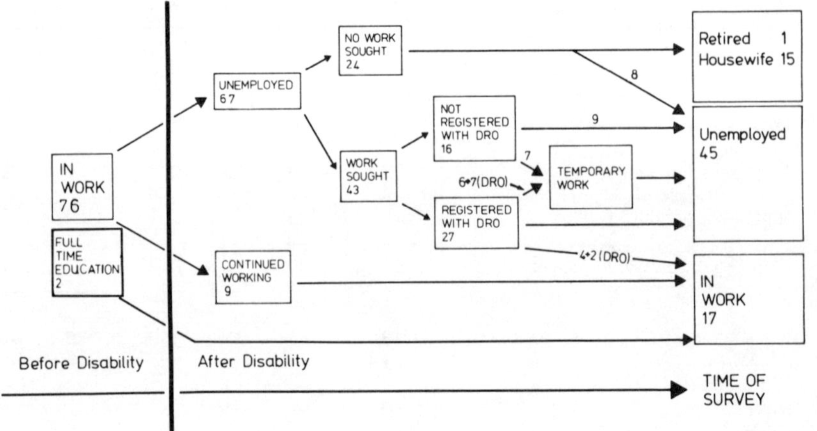

Fig. 10 A flow diagram to indicate the changes in employment of the 76 patients who were in work before the onset of their disability, together with 2 patients who had been in full-time education and later became employed. Note that 16 (37%) of those who had sought work after becoming unemployed were never registered with a DRO.

who had given up work outside the home, and 1 additional retirement. Forty-five of the group were unemployed or unfit for housework.

Changes in employment and registration with Disablement Resettlement Officers (DRO) after onset of disability As stated above 76 patients were in employment before they became disabled. Only 9 of these were able to remain in the same work continuously. Two others found and maintained jobs upon the completion of full-time education courses. Therefore, 67 patients were at some time unemployed as a result of disability.

Among this group who became unemployed were 24 who never sought further work, mostly because they were unfit or because they were women who were unable to work and to run a home at the same time. Forty-three patients, however, had sought work at some stage since becoming disabled. Twenty-seven of the 43 had registered with a DRO but 16 had never been registered. This is 37 per cent of the total number who had sought work since becoming disabled.

The DRO obtained work for 9 of the registered patients and two of them were still working at the time of the survey. Jobs were offered by a DRO to two other registered patients but the work was refused on the grounds that it was menial and poorly paid. In both instances the work was with firms which specifically employ disabled people. Ten of the registered group obtained jobs for themselves, and four of these were still working at the time of survey. The remaining 8 registered patients never found other work.

There were therefore 6 patients who found alternative work, 2 of them with the help of a DRO, who were among the 17 employed at the time of the survey. All 6 had to change their type of work. Two had previously been in professional jobs and 4 in manual skilled jobs but all became clerical workers.

Among the 16 patients who had sought work but had not registered with a DRO, 7 found work for themselves for a short time although none was employed at the time of the survey. The period of employment was often brief (3 weeks to 3 years), either because the job itself was of a temporary nature or because the patient experienced a physical relapse.

Employment rehabilitation The DRO service arranged for 12 patients (11 men and 1 woman) to attend an Industrial Rehabilitation Unit (IRU) for assessment courses lasting between 6 and 36 weeks (average 10 weeks). Five of these undertook a further course of retraining for which they were sponsored by the Department of Employment: three attended a commercial and secretarial college (24 weeks), one attended a Government Training Centre where he did a computer course (44 weeks), and the fifth took a horticultural training course (40 weeks).

All 5 who went for retraining obtained employment following the completion of their course but for 2 the form of retraining was not relevant to the job. Four of the 7 patients who only attended an IRU also obtained employment. Only two patients of the total group of twelve were still employed at the time of interview.

Care at Home

Support by relatives (Fig. 6b)

All participants were living in their own homes or with relatives. None was living in accommodation designed for the disabled although one bedridden patient and his wife had been allocated a house by the Thistle Foundation in Edinburgh and were waiting to move to that sheltered housing scheme.

Among those who were married (79), the care of the patient at home fell principally on the spouse, although older children also played an important role, particularly where the patient was the mother. Several women depended on a married daughter living nearby to do the shopping, the laundry and to assist with housework. In other households these jobs often fell on the husband when he returned home from work or at the weekend. One severely disabled woman had a teenage daughter who, on leaving school, had remained at home to care for her mother instead of getting a job. In another family the father and 4 children (2 of school age) operated a 'shift' system to attend the mother in order that she should be alone for as little time as possible. In both these instances the patient had no home help and no electronic environmental control aid (such as POSSUM) which might have helped her to have some independence from her family (these aids were recommended: *see* section on Aids).

Of those who were not married (25) 11 were living with their parents and 8 were with other relatives. Only 6 patients (2 men and 4 women) lived entirely alone. The ability of parents and relatives to care for a patient with increasing disability was, however, frequently a problem. In several cases the parents were themselves elderly and in other instances, where a patient had moved to live with a younger relative, there was considerable physical and emotional strain on the whole family. Such was the case for one family where the patient was living with her daughter, son-in-law and 6 grand-children in a 5 apartment tenement flat. In another family 3 sisters, all with MS were being cared for by their brother and sister-in-law.

Community health team support

All patients attended a general practitioner (GP). Eight patients were being seen by their GP at least once a fortnight but the remainder saw a GP on average once a month (16) or less frequently than that (80). Many patients only contacted their GP in order to obtain a regular prescription or for authorisation to receive sickness or invalidity benefit. The initiative for contact was therefore nearly always with the patient rather than the GP. Because of this some patients did not see their GP for several months at a time. For example:

> One patient recorded that although she had called her GP during the week prior to interview she had previously not seen him for over a year. This patient was confined to a wheelchair, was disabled in upper and lower limbs and was doubly incontinent. As a district nurse was visiting her twice weekly it might be supposed that she was receiving adequate support from the community health services, yet she badly needed an electronic environmental control aid (POSSUM) which she could only obtain on the recommendation of a hospital consultant following referral by a GP.

Thirty-seven patients were receiving regular visits from a district nurse at the time of interview and 23 others had on different occasions received help from this service. Weekly visits were being made to 19 patients and daily visits to 7 severely disabled patients who required bathing, catheter changes or dressing of pressure sores. The other patients were visited less frequently, usually for the administration of an injection as part of their treatment by the GP.

Twelve patients were currently undergoing a course of physiotherapy, 8 in their own homes and 4 in a hospital department. Sixty-three others had at some time been given this treatment.

Hospital support

The hospital doctor is responsible not only for clinical management but also for referral to the medical social worker, hospital physiotherapy and occupational therapy departments, chiropody, appliance officer, etc. Thirty of the INS group (60 per cent) were attending the INS regularly for medical follow up. Only 9 (16.5 per cent) of the MS Society members were regularly attending hospital. As stated previously, however, the MS Society members were on average older, had been disabled longer and were more severely disabled. Thus the least disabled group were receiving more hospital support.

Inpatient attendances showed the same discrepancy (INS 29, MS Society 17 respectively in the previous twelve months). These figures are not easy to interpret. Some of the patients admitted to the INS had been taken in to allow investigations to be completed. Five at least of the MS Society members had been admitted to allow relatives to take a holiday. Admission had been to geriatric or other wards as there is a shortage of suitable accommodation for the chronic sick in the West of Scotland.

Social Work Services

Forty-one patients said that they had seen a medical social worker (MSW) and 65 patients said that they had seen a social worker from their local authority social work department (LASW). Twenty-six of these patients had seen both medical and local authority social workers. Twenty-four patients stated that as far as they were aware they had never seen a social worker at any time since they became disabled (Fig. 11).

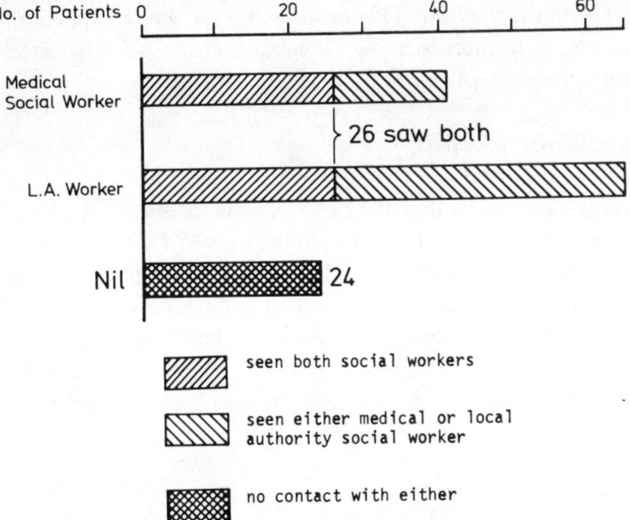

Fig. 11 Contact between patients and medical and local authority social workers at any time since the onset of disability.

Medical Social Worker

Of the 41 patients who said that they had seen an MSW 21 were INS patients and 20 MS Society members. Most of them had first met the social worker either in a hospital ward (24) or an out-patient department (14), although 3 patients had initially been visited in their homes. Twenty-two of the 41 had continued to have contact with an MSW and had seen one at some time during the 12 months preceding the interview. This occurred at the hospital out-patient clinic (15 patients) or at the patients home (5 patients) or both (2 patients). Only 12 of these patients (7 INS, 5 MS Society) however said that they expected to be in further contact. Fifteen patients said that they had only seen an MSW and had not had any additional contact with their local authority social work department. Six of this group were among those who expected further contact with the hospital social work department but the other nine, on ceasing their contact with the MSW, had apparently failed to contact or be put in contact with the local authority social work department and had therefore become 'lost' to social work services in the transition between hospital and home.

Local Authority Social Worker

Sixty-five patients stated that they had had contact with their local authority social work department (22 INS and 43 MS Society). The sources of referral were varied but for 35 (54 per cent) the inital approach to the local social work department was made by the patient himself or a relative. Forty-eight of the patients had seen a social worker and/or local authority occupational therapist during the previous 12 months and 35 of these expected to have further contact with their social work department, usually because they were awaiting the provision of an aid by that department.

Registration of the disabled

Only 19 patients thought that their names were included on a local authority register of disabled people. Two of them had asked for their names to be included on a register and the other 17 believed that a social worker had registered them. Others who had requested practical assistance from their local authority social service departments may have been registered without their knowledge. The MS patients who were registered as disabled did not feel that they benefited in any way from this and were no better informed of services than the rest of the group.

Provision of Services (Fig. 12)

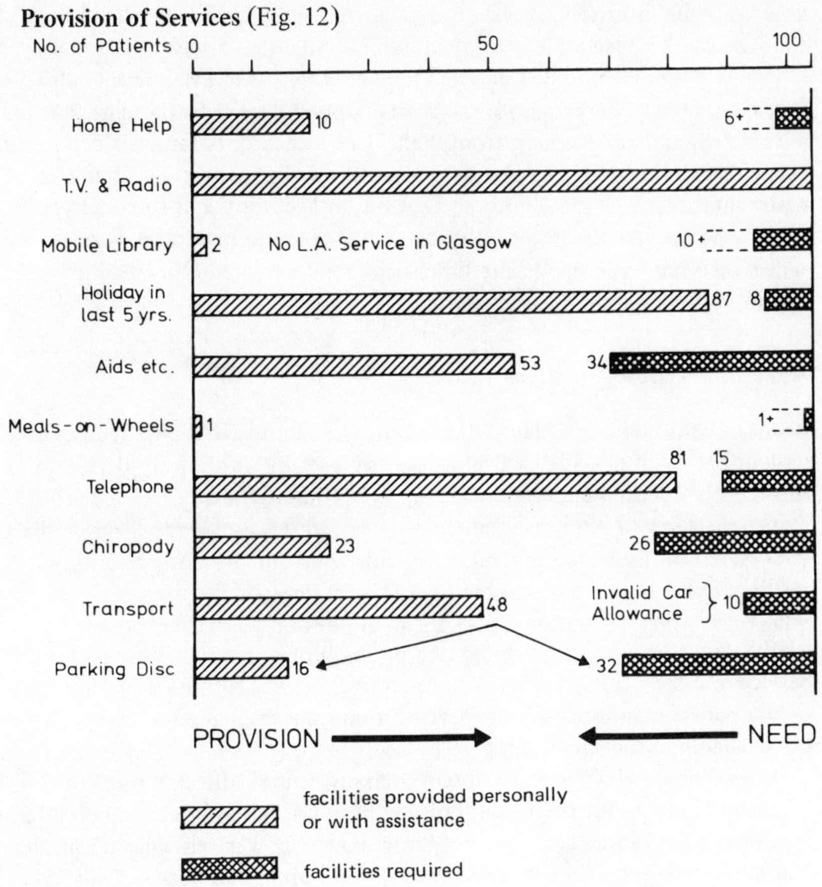

Fig. 12 Provision of some of the facilities covered by the Chronically Sick and Disabled Persons Act (1970). The number of MS patients is indicated on the horizontal scale.

Practical assistance in the home (use of the home-help service)

Although many of the patients were severely disabled, only 20 of them had a local authority home help. Nevertheless, only an additional 6 patients expressed a need for a home help. All of those who had help were women, 3 of them living alone. In 2 cases it was the patients' relative who was provided with a home help as the relative was entirely responsible for the care of the patient. Of those who stated that they needed help 3 had applied to their local authority for the service and were waiting for a home help to be allocated to them. The others were advised to contact their social work department following the interview. Apart from those using the local authority home help service 3 households employed domestic help privately.

A few patients, who had at some time enquired about the home help service, said that they had not made an application as they thought that they would only qualify for help from their local authority (Glasgow Corporation) if they required it daily. Some patients with family members available to assist them felt that a daily home help was unnecessary and too costly. Of those who did use the home help service, 10 received help on 6 days per week and 8 on 5 days per week. The time spent by the home help with the patient varied between 2 and 4 hours per day.

Wireless, television and library services

Every patient had a television set at home and all but five had a radio. One patient had been provided with his television set by a voluntary organisation through the recommendation of an Army Welfare Officer.

The majority of patients made little use of library services because either they were not interested in reading or had visual impairment preventing reading. Some patients were able to visit local libraries themselves or ask relatives or friends to bring books for them, but only 2 patients made use of a voluntary home library service: one by the Womens Royal Voluntary Service and the other by a local community centre. Ten others said that they would use a mobile library service if one was available but this was not available in the survey area.

A few patients had tried to obtain "talking books" through the Royal National Institute for the Blind, but had been unsuccessful as they could not be classified as blind. They did not know that they were eligible to join the National Listening Library which caters for all other handicaps.

Recreational and educational facilities

Fourteen patients attended day centres for the disabled for a whole or part of a day each week. Six of them went to recreational centres run by local authority social service departments and 7 to centres run by the Cripple League, a voluntary organisation. One patient attended a further education day centre for the disabled which was annexed to a college of further education and provided practical tuition in handcrafts.

Transport

Where patients required transport to attend day centres this was provided by the local authority or voluntary organisation concerned with the centre. No patient was provided with transport organised by the local authority for any other purpose. Societies, particularly the MS Society, sometimes arranged transport for their patient members to and from their meetings but this was often by planning for members with cars to convey those without cars.

Provision of vehicles

Twenty patients possessed vehicles of their own. Five had normal cars with manual gears and foot control, 3 had cars which had been adapted to hand controls and 12 had three-wheeler invalid vehicles. All hand-controlled cars had been converted with the aid of grants received from the Department of Health and Social Security and the three-wheelers were provided free of charge by the Department. There were 28 further patients with access to a car for transport. For all but one this was a vehicle privately owned and run by another member of the family. One MS patient, who had formerly been in the Armed Forces, had been provided by the Army with a "mini" especially for his use to be driven by his son. Twenty-five patients said that they could still travel by public transport if necessary and this satisfied their needs. Ten patients expressed a need for an invalid or adapted vehicle because they could no longer drive an ordinary car and found travel by public transport impossible. Two of these patients were waiting to hear the result of their application for a vehicle. Three other patients were eligible at the time of survey for a hand-controlled car as their spouses were also disabled. One of these 3 already possessed a three-wheeler invalid vehicle, but the couple had never been advised that they could apply for a car instead. Their general practitioner was contacted following the interview and an application was made by him on their behalf.

Another man in full employment and fit to drive a special vehicle was relying on colleagues to transport him to and from work. He had been told by his general practitioner that he would not qualify for an invalid vehicle. Following the interview the patient again approached his doctor about applying for a vehicle, but was told (wrongly) that the application would have to be made by a hospital consultant. On querying this with the local centre for issuing vehicles the patient was informed that it was incorrect and that a general practitioner's referral was acceptable. Eight months later, however, an application had still not been made on the patient's behalf. His wife's comment was: 'We have been made to feel that we shouldn't be making such requests'.

Two other patients, one man and one woman, who were not employed, felt that if they had transport they could realistically look for employment. At the time of interview neither of them was eligible for a special vehicle until employment had been found but it was later possible for them to apply for a mobility allowance. Finally, 2 patients who were finding difficulty in driving their ordinary cars were advised at the time of the interview to apply for a grant towards conversion to hand-controls. They subsequently applied through a hospital doctor and were successful.

Parking discs

The discs are issued by local traffic authorities and permit unlimited parking in meter and authorised parking zones, as well as access in pedestrian precincts and limited waiting time in restricted areas. Only 16 people possessed parking discs to be displayed on the window screen of a car driven by a disabled driver or used by a disabled passenger. Eleven were disabled drivers and 5 were disabled passengers. Thirty-two other patients could have claimed a disc, but 9 knew nothing about them and the rest had never bothered to acquire one. Nine drivers who were definitely disabled did not have discs. Six of these owned three-wheelers and felt that the vehicle alone was sufficient to indicate to traffic wardens and police that the driver was disabled. However, 2 owned ordinary cars and a third had a hand-controlled car which could not be identified as belonging to a disabled person.

Aids and alterations to the home

Fifty-three patients were using aids in their home or had made some structural alteration to their house in order to facilitate mobility. Aids which were used ranged from bath seats and hand rails to a hydraulic hoist and an adjustable tilting bed. The most common alterations and additions to the house were the widening of doorways and construction of ramps and stair rails. At the time of interview 10 patients were awaiting the result of applications made to their local authority for aids. There were 24 patients, however, who had not applied for aids but who were found to require them. Some of these patients stated a need for specific aids or house alterations but many did not know about the basic aids for the bathroom and kitchen, nor that these could be obtained through their local authority social work department. Often the provision of small aids, such as a bath seat and hand rail, or some minor installation such as a ramp, would have given the patient greater confidence and independence in the home. For example one patient in a wheelchair was unable to go into her garden unaided for want of a ramp over 2 steps. Nine of the group requiring aids stated that they had previously had contact with an LASW and 8 with an MSW. The remaining 7 said that they had never seen any social worker either at home or in hospital.

Of those patients who already possessed aids many had obtained them through their local authority but some were reluctant to ask for assistance, prefering to buy the aid themselves in order to avoid a means test and the possibility of a long wait while their application was considered. Examples of patients who had been kept waiting for aids or alterations were numerous. In some instances the time was a matter of weeks but for a few patients it was months or even years, by which time the aid originally required might be inadequate if disability had progressed. For example one patient who had requested a ramp from the local authority did not know 6 months later whether or not this was to be provided. Another patient had been assessed for a bath rail by a local authority occupational therapist but was still without a rail 2 years later. A third patient had waited 3 years for work to begin on building a downstairs bathroom in her farm house, which was leased from the local authority. Long delays, repeated attempts to obtain aids, and promises of visits by social workers to patients which were never fulfilled, all added to the frustrations recorded by the patients who were interviewed. Confusion also arose over the respective roles of the social worker and the occupational therapist, particularly those working for the local authority social work department. Many patients were not sure who had been to see them or why they had been visited by more than one person. It would appear, moreover, that such confusion was not confined to the minds of the patients and their relatives as there was evidence of complete breakdown of communication within the Glasgow Social Work Department:

The general practitioner of a severely disabled, bed bound patient wrote to Glasgow Social Work department to ask if a mechanical hoist could be provided. He received a letter of acknowledgement yet when the patient's husband followed up the request social workers and occupational therapists claimed no knowledge of it. When the patient's husband tried to telephone the head occupational therapist for the city he was told that she was intending to visit the patient: she did so four weeks later, after a second telephone call from the husband. The occupational therapist stated that she had no knowledge of the original application for the hoist or of the husband's previous telephone call. The hoist was provided for the patient the following week, 18 weeks after the original application had been made by the general practitioner.

Some of the more expensive aids such as a patient controlled electronic support system (e.g. POSSUM, Possum Controls Ltd.) are provided by the Scottish Home & Health Department on the recommendation and report of a consultant physician. At the time of interview no patient had such a control system although there were several who could have used one to their advantage. Shortly after all the interviews had been completed three patients were referred direct to manufacturers, Possum Controls Ltd., who had asked for information on patients who might be in need of electronic aids. All three patients were severely disabled and by the time that the POSSUM aid became available to them two of the three had died.

The third patient was a woman of 51 years who had been disabled for 16 years and in a wheelchair for 7 years. She had no use of her lower limbs, limited movement only of arms and hands and was doubly incontinent. She had last attended a hospital 14 years ago and had only been seen by her general practitioner once in the 12 months preceding the interview. Although this patient had previously been provided with some simple aids by her local authority and had seen a social worker in the last 6 months no assessment had ever been made for a POSSUM aid. The patient was subsequently provided with a Possum-Link home environment control system through which she was able to operate the front door, an alarm, the television, fire and lights.

Holidays

Eighty-seven of the MS patients had had a holiday of at least a week during the last 5 years. Four patients had obtained a holiday with the help of their local authority, 17 had been to MS Society holiday homes and 2 others had arranged their holiday through the Red Cross Society and Baptist Missionary Society respectively. Seventeen patients had therefore not had a holiday during the last 5 years. Eight of these said that they would particularly like a holiday but felt unable, because of their disability, to stay in a hotel or guest house. None of them knew of special publications which give information about holidays for the disabled nor were they aware that they could ask their local authorities for assistance. Six of the 8 patients who wanted a holiday were MS Society members who knew that the Society ran a Holiday Home in Scotland for its members, but none had investigated the possibility of visiting the home.

Meals-on-wheels

At the time of the survey one married woman, whose husband was working, received meals-on-wheels three days per week. One other patient, a man living alone, said that he would welcome the provision of some meals. He was in touch with a social worker but the idea of applying for this service had never been suggested to him.

Telephone

Twenty-three patients had no direct access to a telephone. Of the 81 households which possessed a telephone only two had received some financial aid towards the installation costs. Both had been given grants by the MS Society and one of these had received an additional grant from their local authority. This was the only example of financial assistance being given by a local authority under the provision of Section 2(1)(h) of the Chronically Sick and Disabled Persons Act. Fifteen of the 23 who did not have a telephone expressed a pressing need for one and 7 of these had already applied to their local authority for financial help. Three had had their application for a grant approved by their local authority although none of these had yet had a telephone installed. Three others had made applications which had been rejected prior to the introduction of the Chronically Sick and Disabled Persons (Scotland) Act (1972). They were therefore advised to re-apply. Each spent part of the day alone at home; two were in wheelchairs and the other had only limited mobility (sticks and a leg caliper).

One patient had obtained an item of special equipment supplied by the

Post Office to aid disabled people to use their telephones more easily. This patient was unable to use a telephone dial and had obtained a 'Sender 1' which, by slight pressure on a button, put him in direct contact with the operator in order to obtain calls. Several other patients with telephones would have benefited from a similar aid.

Table 4: Housing of MS patients (LA: Local Authority)

Housing adequate for disability		
moved house because of disability		
LA	32	
private householders	5	
purpose built accommodation	NIL	
remained in original accommodation	38	
		75
Housing unsuitable for disability		
applied to LA for rehousing	11	
not applied for rehousing		
LA tenants	10	
private householders	8	
		29
		104

Housing

Sixty-eight of the patients were living in local authority houses or flats, 30 in privately owned homes and 6 in rented accommodation. No patient had been provided with a purpose-built house or was living in special accommodation for the disabled although one patient and his wife were about to move to the Thistle Foundation sheltered housing scheme for disabled families in Edinburgh.

Thirty-seven people had moved house because of their disability, 32 of them having been re-housed by their local authority. A further 11 had applied to their local authority to be re-housed, but were still waiting for a house to be allocated to them. Re-housing was usually required because the patient lived one or more storeys up in a tenement building and experienced considerable difficulty in getting out. Three wheelchair users were confined to their houses unless relatives or friends carried them up and down the stairs. They had been waiting to be re-housed for 2½ years, 3 years and 4 years respectively. Some patients could negotiate stairs unaided, but an application for re-housing had been made in anticipation of further physical deterioration. Re-housing might also be indicated if the bathroom was inaccessible to a wheelchair or there were stairs to the bedroom, bathroom or toilet.

In addition to those patients who had applied for re-housing 18 further patients were found to be living in accommodation which, at the time of the survey, was unsuitable for their degree of disability. For example one patient had to be carried up and down stairs by her husband; another could still just negotiate the stairs, but only on her hands and knees; a third could no longer be carried by his elderly father and was, therefore, reduced to sleeping on a sofa downstairs, to using a commode and being bed-bathed. These and other patients seldom, if ever, left their homes as their disability had progressed to a stage which made the effort required to go out too great. One woman stated that she had not been out for four years and one man said that in the last two years the only time he had left his house was to be taken by ambulance to hospital. Despite such difficulties several families did not intend to seek alternative housing. This applied to some who owned their own homes or felt that they received valuable physical help and emotional support from neighbours. Some of the less disabled patients may have been reluctant to face the possibility that their condition could deteriorate further but there were several patients who had never had the possibility of re-housing discussed with them either by a general practitioner, hospital doctor or social worker.

Chiropody

A domiciliary chiropody service is available through the National Health Service in the area covered by the survey. Twenty-three patients were either using this service or visiting a chiropodist at a local centre, but there were 26 severely disabled patients (20 MS Society and 6 INS) who said that they would welcome domiciliary chiropody but who did not know that such a service was available.

Table 5: The sources from which MS patients received the major part of their income.

Income	*No. of Patients*
occupation	17
invalidity benefit	35
sickness benefit	2
pension	14
financial support from relative	36
	104

Financial support

The patients were asked which sources provided the major part of their regular income (Table 5). Seventeen earned an income from their occupation. The remainder of the group were not working. Thirty-five received invalidity benefit and for 14 this was the only form of income, although it was some times supplemented by an allowance towards rent or a special diet. The other 21 received occupational pensions and/or attendance allowances in addition. Two patients who had recently stopped work were drawing sickness benefit. A further 14 patients received an occupational or state pension as their main source of income. The remaining 36 patients who were not working relied on financial support from a relative. Many of these were married women dependent on their husbands, although 19 of the group received an attendance allowance in their own right.

Attendance allowance (Table 6)

At the time of the survey 35 patients were receiving an attendance allowance. Twenty-one of these had a full attendance allowance and 14 had a partial attendance allowance. A further 16 patients (10 MS Society, 6 INS) were considered to be eligible and were advised to apply for one. Two of them had previously had an application for the full attendance allowance rejected and they were therefore advised to reapply for the partial allowance. Eleven of them were no longer being followed up by a hospital doctor. Ten of the patients who were advised to apply for an allowance were successful. Two applicants were turned down but both have requested a review. Three others have not yet heard the result of their applications and only one patient decided not to apply at all. One patient, an MS Society member, who was advised at the time of interview to apply for an allowance, had recourse to the full appeal procedure after her claim was twice rejected. The MS Society helped her to make her appeal which was finally accepted.

Table 6: Patients receiving the attendance allowance at the time of survey and the results of applications made following interview.

Attendance allowance	Multiple Sclerosis Society	Institute of Neurological Sciences	Total
Receiving allowance at survey	26	9	35
full	17	4	
partial	9	5	
Advised to apply	10	6	16
No hospital follow-up	7	4	11
Application successful	5	5	10
Application not made	1	–	1
Pending	4	1	5

Table continued over

Note:
1. 16 (46% of those with allowance) were not receiving an allowance but were advised to apply
2. 11 of these patients no longer have hospital follow-up
3. High success rate following advice to apply (63% so far).
4. This indicates need for regular assessment.

Voluntary Organisations for the Disabled

Sixty-six patients belonged to an organisation concerned with disability. Fifty-four of these were members of the MS Society. Other organisations to which patients belonged included the Cripple League, Disabled Drivers Association, Disablement Income Group, as well as local clubs for the disabled. Several of the patients belonged to more than one of these. A few patients had learned of the existence of such societies from a doctor (9) or social worker (8) but the remainder (49) had only heard by chance through a friend or relative, a fellow patient or through the media.

Multiple Sclerosis Society

Of the 54 patients who were members of the MS Society 37 said that they regularly attended the meetings which were held at their local branch. Some were too disabled to attend and others lacked confidence, believing that physical problems such as frequency of micturition would cause them embarrassment. Most of those who did not attend meetings, however, stated that they had no wish to do so and that they had joined the Society for other reasons, for example to obtain the quarterly magazine, which contains much helpful information.

Discussion

Incidence of Multiple Sclerosis

It is probable that MS affects about 60 per 100,000 of the U.K. population (McAlpine *et al.*, 1972; McAlpine, 1973). The incidence in Scotland and Northern Ireland is slightly higher than in England and Wales (Allison, 1963). Epidemiology in other countries has also been studied extensively (McAlpine *et al.*, 1972; U.S. Advisory Commission on MS, 1974; Dean, 1975).

A survey of an urban population in which an attempt was made to identify all disabled people drew attention to the great preponderance of diseases of the central nervous system amongst respondents falling into the most severe category of disablement (Fryers, Banning and Newton, 1974). In the total population (130,530) of the city of Salford, Lancashire, 2643 disabled people were identified and 29 of these suffered from MS (1:4,500). Ten of these were in the most severely disabled group and MS was one of the five common neurological disorders causing at least this amount of severe disability. As MS is, however, thought to be more common in the community it may be that that survey, although identifying major disability, did not indicate the true incidence of the disease, many patients with little or no continuing disability perhaps not even knowing their diagnosis. These and other contributory factors in the difficulties of interpretation of prevalence rates are emphasized in the report of the U.S. National Advisory Commission on MS (1974) which recommended increased research because of the extent of disability which the disease causes.

Comparison with other reported groups

The characteristics of the disease in the group approximated to those reported elsewhere. MS tends to occur more frequently in women than in men. The average sex ratio in several series of studies was 1:1.7, male: female (McAlpine *et al.*, 1972). In this survey the male/female ratio was 1:1.17, the MS Society members being in the ratio 1: 2.18. Another survey which included patient members of the MS Society in New Zealand (McCallum, 1973) found a higher proportion of females among the society members and suggested that this could be attributed to a greater female interest in society membership. In the present survey most of the patients were aged between 40 and 60 years and the mean age of onset was 30–40 years. Similar observations were reported in the New Zealand survey. The age of onset is sometimes said to be more frequently 20–30 years (Panelius, 1969). In our survey the majority had been disabled for up to 20 years but 17 (16%) had been disabled for between 20 and 40 years. This finding is in keeping with recent recognition that the disorder may be of long duration and frequently benign for many years (Percy *et al.*, 1971; Editorial, British Medical Journal, 1972). The survey by Percy *et al.*, carried out in Rochester, Minnesota showed a 25 year survival rate of 74% compared with 86% expected survival (Percy *et al.*, 1971).

The effect of MS upon marital relations was not examined in detail. Only 4 of 79 marriages had broken down after the development of the disease, implying that our patients had considerable marital support and stability. These figures are slightly better than those from other surveys, 8 out of 69 marriages having failed in the New Zealand survey (McCallum, 1973) and 7 out of 45 marriages in a London borough (Stevens, 1974). MS may cause impotence in the male (Cartlidge, 1972) but the extent of this problem and its affect on marital relations was not examined. The sexual and emotional needs of the handicapped have recently been reviewed by Greengross (1976).

Multiple Sclerosis is one of the major neurological causes of severe disability in the community (Fryers *et al.*, 1974). The extent of disability among the patients in this study was in keeping with this observation as 99 of the patients had difficulty with walking. In the New Zealand series of McCallum 32 out of 100 were bedfast or confined to a chair, compared with 34 in our series, implying comparability of the two groups. Our group and that in New Zealand probably contained a high proportion of seriously affected patients thereby exaggerating the impression that severe disability occurs rapidly. Two thirds of the survivors diagnosed in one area (Rochester, Minnesota) were ambulant 25 years after diagnosis (Percy *et al.*, 1971). In our group 47 patients experienced depression and 23 complained of intellectual deterioration. In a psychiatric study of 108 patients with mild to severe physical disability it was found that two thirds of MS patients had intellectual deterioration and a quarter were depressed (Surridge, 1969). No formal psychiatric assessment of our patients was made but our findings confirm that depression and intellectual deterioration are of frequent occurrence although earlier workers had failed to recognise that these symptoms were extensive (Cottrell and Wilson, 1927).

Employment

At the time of the survey only 17 patients were employed (full-time) while

45 had become unemployed as a result of disability. A similar low rate of employment among MS patients was found in New Zealand (McCallum, 1973) where 16 out of 100 patients were working and 52 were unemployed. Cessation of work does not, however, tend to be abrupt and many of those interviewed had been able to hold their jobs for several years until disability became too severe. Twenty-two had been able to work intermittently in other jobs while being disabled but this tended to necessitate a change of occupation, often to lower status work with a reduced income. For example:

> one patient who had been a sheet metal worker was reduced to sweeping a factory floor; another who had been a long distance lorry driver moved to be a garage fuel pump attendant, and then a lavatory attendant before giving up work.

In such circumstances the patient has little incentive to continue working. A further problem in maintaining employment is that the MS patient tends to be viewed as a 'poor risk' by employers for the nature of MS oftens means periods of absenteeism from work due to relapses.

The assistance of a DRO was found to be helpful to some patients and 9 obtained jobs as a result of this service although this was only a third of those who had registered. There were, however, sixteen patients (37 per cent of those who at one time were seeking work) who had never registered with a DRO and who might have benefited from the service. Advice on employment may be helpful to the patient, even in the early stages of disability. The need for this for MS patients was pointed out by Brown (1969) and McCallum (1973) for groups in the U.S.A. and New Zealand respectively. The failure of the British DRO service to be in contact with some disabled patients who might have benefited from help was a finding in a survey of patients with paraplegia in 1971/2 (Johnson and Johnson, 1972, 1973) in the same region as the present study. Twenty-three out of 44 of the patients in the paraplegic group who were potentially employable had not seen a DRO.

Care at home

Support by relatives

Only 6 (6 per cent) of the patients interviewed in the survey were living alone. This proportion is considerably lower than that found in the Salford survey (27.3 per cent) or the national survey of handicapped and impaired (21 per cent) (Buckle, 1971; Harris, 1971). Those surveys, however, included all types of handicap. In a survey of 62 patients disabled by MS and other neurological diseases (Stevens, 1974) in which the majority (45) suffered from MS, only 5 (8 per cent) lived alone. These results would suggest that the disabilities associated with MS lead to a greater degree of dependence among patients with this disorder. It may also be that the slow progression of the disease in many patients allows relatives to become adjusted to problems without family disruption.

Support by the Community Health team and hospital doctors

The patients received much support from General Practitioners. There is however, so little treatment that can be given for the disorder that follow-up was intermittent and information about social support would therefore be similarly restricted. In our examination of hospital outpatient attendances we found that there was more follow-up given to patients who were on average the less disabled in the total group. The present system of medical care, therefore, places the severely disabled at a considerable disadvantage.

There was no common policy about informing patients of the cause of their disability. We found that all patients who knew their diagnosis were glad to do so and conclude that as a broad rule all patients who have *continuing* disability from MS should have the diagnosis named and discussed with them and their closest relative.

Social work services

In hospital a medical social work service is usually available to patients who attend either as in-patients or out-patients. It might be expected that these would be the more seriously disabled patients but the present survey showed that the more disabled group of patients (MS Society members) had less hospital follow-up than the less disabled group (INS patients). Therefore those patients attending hospital and having access to medical social workers were not necessarily those most in need of social work support and services (see previous section).

A large number of patients had apparently not seen any social worker during the course of their disability. Others (15) had seen a MSW but were not in contact with the Social Service Department of their local authority from which many of the home services for disabled people are organised. It could be argued that those who were not in touch with a social work department were able to organise their own requirements independently but this was not found to be correct and more often these patients were less well informed about the services available and how to apply for them. For example of 24 patients who were found to be in need of aids in the home 7 had never seen a social worker and the remainder had had no recent contact with social work services. Seven patients who stated a need for a telephone had no contact with their local authority social service department.

However, contact between the patient and the social service departments still did not necessarily ensure that the patient would be adequately informed of facilities available to him. It appeared that social workers were failing to examine the full range of needs of the disabled patients and that some of the social workers themselves lacked knowledge of the services available through their own departments as well as through other departments and agencies. For example, of 8 patients requiring advice about holidays for the disabled 5 had seen a social worker within the 6 months prior to the survey but had never had this topic discussed. Eighteen of the 26 patients who stated a need for chiropody had seen a social worker in the previous 12 months but had not been told of the domiciliary chiropody service.

The lack of information among patients of financial benefits available to them, in particular the attendance allowance, was of more serious consequence.

Attendance allowance

A person may claim this allowance from the department of Health & Social Security if for at least 6 months he has been so disabled as to require from another person:

(a) by day = i. frequent attention throughout the day in connection with his bodily functions, or
ii. continual supervision throughout the day in order to avoid substantial danger to himself or others and/or

(b) by night = i. prolonged or repeated attention during the night in connection with his bodily functions, or
ii. continual supervision throughout the night in order to avoid substantial danger to himself or others.

The application includes a medical report by a doctor, usually the patients general practitioner, and in some instances the patient will also be examined by a doctor nominated by the Attendance Allowance Board. Applicants are not means tested, but are assessed solely on their disability. Two levels of grant are available: the partial attendance allowance is awarded to patients who require someone in attendance either by day or night, and the full attendance allowance is given to those who meet both the day and the night conditions. When granted, the allowance is backdated to the date of application. It is tax free and is not regarded as a source of income for the purposes of most means tests for other support.

A claimant who is refused on his first application has the right to apply for a review within three months and, if successful, payments are backdated to the date of the original application. If the applicant is again refused a final appeal may be made to the National Insurance Commissioners.

At the time of the interview 35 patients were receiving an attendance allowance but in the view of the interviewer an additional 16 patients had good cause to apply for the allowance (Table 5). Twelve of the 16 had seen a social worker in the previous 12 months but had not been advised to make an application. Yet 10 of the group succeeded in obtaining an attendance allowance when they applied for one immediately after the survey. These findings indicate failure on the part of social workers to ensure that patients were receiving available financial benefits or that they at least knew how to apply for such benefits and the basis on which cash was granted. It was the impression of the interviewer that patients would not necessarily act on written information which they received unless this was followed up by a verbal explanation. For example several patients had not realised that the attendance allowance was not means tested. They had not applied for fear of a means test because they felt that their level of income would exclude them, or because they were already receiving a supplementary pension and thought that this would disqualify them from further benefits. Other patients were reluctant to apply for the allowance as they did not believe themselves to be sufficiently disabled. They needed the advice of a social worker or doctor who could assess their degree of disability and compare them with other patients already receiving the allowance. Social work follow-up was shown to be necessary even among those who were advised to apply for an attendance allowance at the time of interview. The interviewer acted on behalf of 2 of the patients by arranging for application forms to be sent to them from the Department of Health and Social Security. Two others were prompted to make applications by a follow-up telephone call from the interviewer and three patients were encouraged to apply for reviews when their initial applications were rejected. Such measures require a period of intensive follow-up work by the social worker. By dealing with practical matters and helping to ease any financial strain the social worker may then find him or herself better able to assist the patient and his family in coping with emotional problems associated with disability. Moreover if the patient and his relatives can define an area in which they received positive assistance from a social worker they may be more willing to approach the social services themselves at a future date if need arises.

Registration of the disabled

Section 1 of the Chronically Sick and Disabled Persons Act (1970) which was extended to Scotland in the Chronically Sick and Disabled Persons (Scotland) Act (1972) requires that local authorities must assess the numbers and needs of chronically sick and disabled persons in their area. In doing this, social service departments are expected to compile a comprehensive register of their disabled. The register should not, however, be an end itself but should facilitate the dissemination of information to the disabled and efficient management of their needs.

In the present survey only 19 MS patients believed that their names were included on a local authority register of the disabled and there was no evidence that Section 1 of the Acts was being implemented. Those patients who were registered had not found this to bring any benefits and it was more likely that the provision of services led to the registration of the patient rather than vice versa. At the present time the only certain advantage arising out of registration is that it is used by local authorities as the basis for awarding rent rebates and higher needs allowances to disabled people (Department of Health and Social Security Circular 43, 1972), (Lynes, 1972).

To extend this and make registration a pre-requisite for acquiring other services, however, might cause antipathy among the disabled. Some people do not wish their names to be included in registers as this represents categorisation and a threat to their independence. They may also fear loss of confidentiality in their dealings with social and medical workers, wondering to whom and for what purposes the register is made available. In the national survey of handicapped and impaired 70 per cent of the respondents, who did not know previously about registration, said that they would not wish to be registered (Harris, 1971). On the other hand registration will be seen to be meaningful and therefore more acceptable if:

1. as a result of registration disabled people are kept informed of services and benefits available,

2. the disabled receive some form of periodic follow-up and reassessment,

3. disabled persons are informed of the purpose of the register and agree to their names being added.

These conclusions are discussed later in this report.

Provision of Services

Section 2, of the Chronically Sick and Disabled Persons Act (1970), and that of Scotland (1972) list the following amenities which should be available to the disabled:

(a) Practical assistance in the home
(b) Wireless, television, library or similar recreational facilities
(c) Lectures, games, outings, recreational facilities outside the home and educational facilities
(d) Assistance in travelling to use services outside the home.
(e) Assistance with home adaptations
(f) Holiday facilities
(g) Meals at home or elsewhere
(h) Telephone or any special equipment necessary for its use

Section 3 of the Act details local authorities responsibilities about housing and Section 19 lays down the need for chiropody for the disabled.

Practical assistance in the home (Home helps)

The local authority home help service provides support for patients by assisting disabled housewives to run their homes and providing a person to be in attendance for at least part of the day. This is particularly valuable for patients whose disability imposes an accident risk. As well as basic house cleaning, a home help is allowed to carry out shopping, laundering and the preparation of meals. The cost of the service to the patient is means related. There is a minimum charge and since 1973 the service has been provided free to those receiving Supplementary Benefit. For those needing help in the home, and especially those patients receiving an attendance allowance, the cost should not be prohibitive.

Local authority divisions in the survey area do not operate any restrictions on the number of days per week on which the home help service may be provided and as far as possible the service attempts to meet the needs of the client. The patients in Glasgow who thought that they could only obtain the home help service if they required it every day were misinformed about current practice. The Glasgow service is available from a minimum of 2 hours to a maximum of 38 hours per week. Possibly a more significant factor determining reluctance to apply for a home help is the socially unacceptable idea of employing domestic help, however nominal the charge. This feeling was voiced by one patient who withdrew her application after being allocated a home help who lived in the same street.

Wireless, television and library

All patients in the survey had wireless and/or television at home and there was no need for further provision. There was, however, a small demand for a home library service, which at present only operates in rural localities. Although many patients had difficulty in handling books or had visual impairment which hampered reading no one was a member of the National Listening Library or knew about it.

The National Listening Library was started in 1972 for those unable to read or handle a book in the ordinary way but who do not qualify for the similar service run by the Royal National Institute for the Blind (R.N.I.B.). The cost of the service is high (£12 annual membership and £39.60 to buy the machine (June, 1976), compared with the R.N.I.B. annual subscription of £6 which covers everything including hire of a machine). However, patients with low incomes should be able to apply under Section 2(b) of the Acts to their local authority for a grant towards joining the library.

Recreational and educational facilities

The facilities in the area included recreational day centres and a further education day centre, an annex of Langside College. These were much appreciated by the patients.

Assistance with transport

Ten patients who were no longer able to drive an ordinary car required invalid vehicles or help towards adapting cars for their use. Five of them did not know they were eligible for such help and it was apparent that medical practitioners were not well informed about the criteria for eligibility or the method of application for invalid vehicles. The patients in the survey who were receiving assistance with personal transport had obtained either an invalid vehicle or a private car allowance.

Until July 1976 the single seater, 3–wheel *invalid car* 'tricycle' was available to severely and permanently disabled people or to those whose disability was less severe but who required transport to and from full-time work. The vehicle was provided, maintained and insured by the Department of Health and Social Security. In July 1976 the Government announced its intention to phase out the use of tricycles over the next five years but no plans have been announced for an alternative vehicle. No tricycles are being issued to new applicants. Until January 1976 *modified four–wheel cars* (usually a 'mini') were provided to disabled people in exceptional circumstances, for example to disabled mothers with young children or to two disabled relatives in the same household. This scheme has now ceased. A *private car allowance* of £100 per annum for maintaining a private vehicle was available as an alternative to provision of an invalid tricycle. Since the survey was completed the *Mobility Allowance* has been introduced, to take the place of the invalid tricycle and the private car allowance (July 1976). This is a weekly allowance available to severely disabled people aged between 5 years and retirement age (60 years for women, 65 years for men). The current rate of the allowance (October 1976) is £5 per week (£260 per annum) and the Government has announced its intention to increase the rate by £2 per week in November 1977.

The advantage of the mobility allowance is that it offers help to both disabled drivers and non-drivers. It is therefore of particular value to disabled people who are unable to drive and who have not previously received any Government help towards mobility. There are, however, disadvantages to the scheme:

i. The medical conditions of eligibility for the mobility allowance are limiting. A claimant must be virtually unable to walk and yet must be sufficiently mobile to make use of the allowance. In a progressive disorder such as multiple sclerosis with its common pattern of exacerbations and remissions a patient may fluctuate between an eligible and non-eligible condition and therefore be difficult to assess.
ii. The mobility allowance is taxable.
iii. Those receiving the mobility allowance are required to pay vehicle excise duty if they own a car. Previously invalid tricycle owners and recipients of the private car allowance were exempt from payment.
iv. The mobility allowance ceases at retirement age.

Moreover, although the Mobility Allowance is to replace the Government issue of invalid vehicles it is nowhere near the same financial value. The mobility allowance is barely sufficient to maintain a car, let alone to buy one and there is anxiety that tricycle drivers are therefore going to be denied the degree of mobility which they have previously experienced. A leading article in *The Times* at the time of the announcement of the Government's plans, suggested that 'today's tricycle drivers are likely to be driven from the road' as these were the 'drivers who, almost by definition, have been unable to afford the four-wheeled cars they would prefer' (*The Times* leader 21st July 1976). A spokesman for the Invalid Tricycle Action Group said that many disabled drivers would have to give up their jobs because they would no longer be able to afford to get to work (report in *The Times,* 27th July 1976).

Most of the patients interviewed in this survey will be eligible to apply for the mobility allowance. There may be some however who are not in contact with a social worker or receiving regular hospital follow-up and may therefore not get to know about the details of the allowance.

The parking disc scheme was only a limited success as many patients were poorly informed.

Assistance with home adaptations

Nearly a quarter (24) of the patients required aids but had not received advice about them. Ten of these patients had had contact with their local authority social work department but had not been referred to occupational therapists. The failure to provide information and referral for occupational therapy assessment for these patients may be due to limited knowledge on the part of some social workers of the aids available for the disabled.

Holiday facilities

Information about holidays was limited. In particular the patients did not know about the financial and other support which may be available from local authorities.

Meals-on-wheels

This service was little used but information about it had not always been given.

Telephone

Under the Act local authorities are empowered to assist a disabled person to obtain a telephone or special equipment for its use. Special telephone equipment for the disabled is available from the G.P.O. and detailed in the Post Office leaflet DLE 550. Only one patient knew about this and had obtained one of the aids. Other patients, particularly those with severe motor disability in their hands and arms, might have benefited from a telephone aid had they known that these were available. The range of aids includes a 'keyphone receiver', an automatic call maker' for those who are unable to use a telephone dial, and a 'lightweight headset' for those unable to hold a handset.

The policy of local authorities over allocating grants towards telephones varies and the interviewer found patients who had been refused help but who were more disabled and isolated than 2 of those who had had their application for a grant approved. A year after the Chronically Sick and

Disabled Persons Act was passed Lanark County Council announced plans to allocate £1000 towards provision of telephones (*Glasgow Herald* 3rd June, 1971) but Glasgow Corporation took until 1973 before launching a pilot scheme to install 100 telephones in the homes of disabled people (*Glasgow Herald* 27th November, 1973).

It was possible that so long as Sections 1 and 2 of the Chronically Sick and Disabled Persons Act (1970) did not apply to Scotland local authorities in this area felt no mandate on them to provide telephones (Johnson and Johnson, 1972, 1973). However, the introduction of the Chronically Sick and Disabled Persons (Scotland) Act, 1972, with its clearer definition of the statutory powers of local authorities in Scotland appears to have been no more effective. There is evidence that at least one local authority in the survey area has not allowed for any grants towards telephones for the disabled in its annual budgets.

One of us was contacted by a social worker from Motherwell who wrote: 'I approached the Director of Social Work regarding a telephone installation but was told that this local authority does not make any provision for this service'. The Acting Town Clerk of Motherwell was asked whether the Burgh of Motherwell intended to give support under the Act. He eventually replied saying that he had not been directly involved in the question of the provision of telephones. He gave details from the Minutes of the Council's Social Work Committee: 'The Town Council would be prepared to finance the provision of telephones for the handicapped if the Secretary of State was prepared to increase substantially the present grant arrangements'. They were, however, informed that there was no arrangement for external aid for the provision of telephones apart from help to a person who was geographically isolated and receiving supplementary benefit. In other cases the costs should be borne by the authority. 'In subsequent years a sum of money was included by the Director of Social Work in his draft estimates for the provision of telephones for the disabled but each year, when the Council considered the demands on their financial resources overall, including the many requirements of the Social Work function, this amount was deleted from the final estimates. It seems clear, therefore, that the Town Council did not make specific provision for the supply of telephones to the disabled'.

A circular issued to local authorities by the Social Work Services Group (5th May, 1972) offering guidelines on the financing of telephones seems to have caused confusion among some authorities and frustration for the patients. The circular made it clear that a grant towards the installation charge and/or continuing assistance towards the rental of a telephone could be met by local authorities. The Post Office will install a telephone for a disabled user at a reduced charge on one of the following conditions:-

(a) The telephone is rented in the name of the Local Authority;
(b) in the name of the beneficiary, with the Local Authority undertaking responsibility for any outstanding telephone accounts;
(c) in the name of the beneficiary, without local authority indemnity but with an initial deposit paid against the first telephone account at the time of installation.

The circular also listed minimum criteria which would entitle an applicant to financial help:-

The applicant should

1. have a *prima facie* need to get in touch with his doctor quickly and would be in danger if left alone unless provided with a telephone;
2. live alone or, if not, be regularly and frequently left alone and be unable in normal weather to leave the house without the help of another person;
3. indicate at least one person willing to be in touch by telephone and, in the view of the authority, need a telephone to avoid isolation;
4. have no family, friends or neighbours generally available and willing and able to help.

This last requirement has made it possible for local authorities to refuse almost every claim for help as there are few people so spacially isolated that they do not have a neighbour to whom they can turn in an emergency. Instances have been reported where the conditions of eligibility were carried to the extreme:

> Social workers in Lanarkshire were told that disabled applicants for a telephone grant would be required to make a list of all the people whom they wished to telephone. Another authority considered issuing disabled residents with whistles to use to summon help.

The guidelines were intended to bring about a degree of uniformity among local authorities in their policy towards making grants for telephones, but the wording of the circular implies a failure to recognise the mental and physical isolation of those who are largely house-bound and the sense of security and independence that can be gained by possessing a telephone. It also emphasises the responsibility of the family towards the disabled patient whereas many would argue that the aim of the community health and social services should be towards increasing the support to relatives in order that disabled people can be more readily and safely accommodated in their own homes.

Housing

The Chronically Sick and Disabled Persons Act, 1970 (Section 3) places a duty on local housing authorities to have regard for the special needs of the disabled and to make provision for them when planning new housing. The results of the present survey show that help was made available by local authorities to adapt existing houses for the convenience of the disabled occupants. In addition most housing authorities possess lists of houses and flats which have been adapted and which may be reallocated to other disabled people in the future. Several patients (32) were rehoused in more suitable ground level accommodation but the process of rehousing was often slow and 11 patients were still waiting to be moved. No one occupied a purpose built house. A survey of Handicapped and Impaired in Great Britain estimated that 3 in 5 adults suffering from impaired mobility were aged 65 years or over and that most lived alone or with one other person (Buckle and Harris, 1971). Therefore some older people can be suitably housed in sheltered schemes for the elderly. In some areas, e.g. East Kilbride, sheltered housing is not reserved solely for the elderly and a proportion may be occupied by handicapped people well under retirement age. However, there was inadequate provision of housing for young handicapped people with families, particularly those in wheelchairs, such as many of the MS patients interviewed in this survey.

The number of purpose built houses for the disabled available in the survey area is Dunbarton 1, Motherwell 4 and Erskine 4. East Kilbride has 11 houses suitable for wheelchair users within sheltered housing schemes. The most recent purpose built houses to be opened were the 4 in Erskine New Town in May 1975. These have been built by the Scottish Special Housing Association and have the following special features:

1. General increase in space standards in accordance with recommendations contained in *Designing for the Disabled* (Goldsmith, 1967)
2. Wide doors and corridors to enable wheelchairs to manoeuvre easily
3. Special W.C. and bathroom fitments e.g. grips, handrails, etc.
4. No steps
5. All door handles, shelves, light switches and power points within reach of wheelchair users
6. Sliding doors between kitchen/livingroom and bedroom/livingroom
7. Low windows, so that wheelchair users can see out
8. (a) Adjustable height for sink, hob unit and work top
   (b) Delivery hatch
   (c) Oven and hob unit separate to enable hob to be adjustable
   (d) Ironing board folded away at low level for wheelchair users
   (e) All cupboards, worktops, shelves, etc., within reach of wheelchair users.

A circular from the Secretary of State for Scotland in May 1975 drew attention to the scarcity of purpose built housing throughout Scotland, particularly for young handicapped people, and strongly recommended

> . . . that in the planning of all sizeable new housing developments in the future, housing authorities should make provision, based on an assessment of need, for some housing for physically handicapped people (Scottish Development Department circular 61, 29th May 1975).

Despite this there appear to be no plans at present for building houses for the disabled in the survey area although most authorities state their intention to consider the need for such housing at a future date.

One of the difficulties of providing specialised houses in the public sector is keeping them continuously occupied by disabled tenants. One local authority Housing Manager stated:

> It would seem to us to be preferable to provide an appropriate range of house types for general family use but which have been designed in such a way as to make their adaptation for handicapped people relatively simple . . . the great difficulty is ensuring that the supply of accommodation is available at the same time as demand, and vice-versa. Unfortunately we have some experiences where this is not the case" (personal communication from the Housing Manager, East Kilbride and Stonehouse Development Corporation).

Chiropody

It has already been noted that ancillary supporting services were often not explained to patients. This also applied to 26 patients who expressed a need for this service.

Current problems in the provision of services

In the previous section upon provision of services we found that many patients lacked forms of support from which they would have benefited. We have shown that part of the failure is due to some patients having inadequate or no contact with social services or other sources of advice and information.

The failure of the social services to meet the needs of many of the patients must not, however, lie only with individual social workers. Other, wider issues affect the provision of social work support for the disabled. These include the following:

1. Social work services lack sufficient resources of money and man-power to provide adequate cover.
2. Local authorities have failed to identify the disabled in their area.
3. There are failures of communication which result in disabled people becoming lost 'to the system'.

These are discussed in this section of the report

Insufficient resources

A report published by the Department of the Environment in 1975 described Glasgow and much of the Strathclyde region as: 'the most deprived area in Britain for housing, unemployment and overcrowding' (Report, Department of Environment, 1975). Conditions which are described in such terms lead to a heavy demand on all local authority services and consequently on the money available to finance them. It has been pointed out by Strathclyde Regional Council that the present government rate support grant is insufficient to meet the particular problems of the region and the Chairman of the Council, Mr Geoffrey Shaw, has stated: It is our responsibility . . . to look for a greater injection of central government funds (*The Times* 16th April, 1975) At the same time local authorities are being asked to curb their spending and in the financial cuts that will arise services for the disabled must undoubtedly suffer. As we have indicated, local authorities may be reluctant to become involved in additonal spending for such items as telephones for the disabled or to include special housing in their redevelopment programmes.

Financial restrictions may also prevent local authorities from employing a full quota of trained social workers and, in addition, there is the problem that an area such as Glasgow may prove unattractive to potential workers.

Glasgow social service officers have repeatedly drawn attention to the shortage of field workers, a 25% shortfall being reported by the previous director of social work for the City (*Glasgow Herald* 4th September, 1973) who commented that incentives were lower for potential workers in Glasgow than in other areas.

Although Glasgow's difficulties are considerable it would be wrong to assume that the problems are confined to its area. There is evidence of a national failure in the uniform provision of services within the budget available. Although it could be argued that inequalities are related to differing numbers of disabled this is not so.

In April 1973, 2½ years after the implementation of the Chronically Sick and Disabled Persons Act, 1970, Mr Jack Ashley, M.P., introduced a motion in the House of Commons deploring the long delay in the implementation of the Act. He referred to a report that 19 local authorities had spent less on the chronically sick and disabled in the last financial year than in the one before, and he asked if the Government was sure that all the money allocated for the disabled was being used for this purpose by the local authorities. The report to which he referred ("The Implementation of the Chronically Sick and Disabled Act 1970", February, 1973), revealed considerable variation between authorities in England and Wales in the provision of services specified in the Act. For example expenditure per annum on home helps varied by a factor of four and expenditure on house adaptations differed between some areas by as much as a factor of 12. Similar disparities were shown between local authorities in the West of Scotland at that time (Johnson and Johnson, 1972, 1973) and it would appear from the present survey that there is still significant variation in the policies adopted by these local authorities towards expenditure on provisions for the disabled.

Failure to identify the disabled

As previously stated, Section 1 of the Chronically Sick and Disabled Persons Act, 1970, which was extended to Scotland in the Chronically Sick and Disabled Persons (Scotland) Act 1972, requires that local authorities must assess the numbers and needs of chronically sick and disabled persons in their areas. In doing this social service departments are expected to compile a comprehensive register of their disabled.

In the present survey only 19 MS patients believed that their names were included on a local authority register of the disabled. Others, who had requested practical assistance from their local social service departments, may have been registered without their knowledge. In either case, however, registration did not appear to result in any attempt at regular, albeit infrequent, follow-up to assess changing needs. Thirty-nine patients (37.5 per cent) were, according to their own statements, unknown to their local authority social service departments. We found that among a group of paraplegics in the same survey area, 18 per cent of the sample were apparently unknown to their local authority social services (Johnson and Johnson, 1973).

The survey on the 'Implementation of the Chronically Sick and Disabled Act' (Report, 1973) found that more than one third of the local authority social service departments in England and Wales had no plans to estimate the number of disabled people in their area. By the time that survey report was published only 370,000 people had been identified as being so significantly handicapped that they needed services. Yet an earlier survey had estimated a total of 1,129,000 people (Harris, 1971).

At the time that the Chronically Sick and Disabled Persons Act became law the Department of Health and Social Security and the Office of Population Censuses produced recommendations for identifying the disabled and a guideline to sampling for local authorities. Some authorities produced well documented surveys: for example Kensington and Chelsea (1972), Newcastle upon Tyne (1972), Preston (1972), Isle of Wight (1972), Salford (1974), but others have been criticised publically for failing to attempt to identify their disabled:

> 'Some authorities have evaded their responsibilities under the Chronically Sick and Disabled Persons Act, 1970, in a way little short of criminal negligence'.
> – Mr. Charles Irving, M.P., addressing a symposium held by the British Association of Social Workers (reported in *The Times* 11th April, 1975)

The results of surveys already carried out point to extensive areas of unknown and unmet need among the disabled in the community. For example in the Isle of Wight 8.4 per cent of households contained a previously unknown disabled resident, while in Newcastle upon Tyne the figure was 18 per cent of households. The Preston survey suggested that over half the estimated number of 4,495 disabled persons in the town were in need of a telephone (quoted by Gregory, 1973).

Only one of the previously existing local authorities in the Strathclyde Region made any attempt to identify its disabled along the lines recommended. In 1972/3 Paisley used volunteers to conduct a house to house survey which revealed that there were 900 elderly house-bound and 430 other physically handicapped people in the town. Following the survey, proposals for a 6 year plan for the expansion of social work in Paisley, costing approximately £4 million, were submitted to the Secretary of State for Scotland. The largest single project was special housing for the disabled. There was also provision to double the number of social workers and the annual expenditure on social work services in Paisley (*Glasgow Herald* 5th February, 1973).

If some local authorities can attempt to identify their disabled in this way, why not others? The most common argument, which was put by directors of social services to Mr Alfred Morris, Under-Secretary of State for the Disabled, in October 1974, is that there is little point in devoting scarce time and man-power to identify people whose needs cannot be met (*The Times,* 23rd October, 1974). There are fears of excessive demand on services and that attempts to identify need would only raise expectations among the disabled that could not be fulfilled. However, it may be that by revealing such inadequacies local authorities gain backing for their claims for more financial aid to be directed towards services for the disabled. This has occurred in Manchester, a city comparable in size to Glasgow, where considerable unknown and unmet need among the disabled was revealed. The social services department gathered information from doctors, dentists, clergy, chemists, medical social workers and members of the city council. In addition information booklets were distributed and publicity was directed to national and local newspapers, national and regional television networks and local radio. As a result 19,000 disabled people were registered between 1971 and 1975. This was four times the previous number of registered chronic sick and disabled in that city whereas nationally the number registered has only slightly more than doubled (*The Times* 26th January, 1976). The figures provided impetus for co-operation between local government departments in the provision of services and have justified the spending of £635,000 between 1971 and 1975 on meeting obligations under Sections 1 and 2 of the Chronically Sick and Disabled Persons Act in Manchester.

Failures of communication

The effectiveness of social work support for the care of the disabled patient living at home frequently depends on communications between health workers and social workers in hospital and in the community. The importance of adequate communication between the services has been stressed by a study of paraplegics in Liverpool which reported 'many failures in communication which resulted in frustration and hazards for the patients and their relations' (Forder, Reti and Silver, 1969).

Our survey has shown that the more disabled group of patients (MS Society members) had less hospital follow-up than the less disabled group (INS patients). Therefore those patients attending hospital and having access to medical social workers were not necessarily those most in need of social work support and services. Even for those patients who attend a hospital clinic referral to a medical social worker usually depends upon the selection by the hospital doctor of patients who need social work help. The patients who are referred to a social worker are more likely to be those who verbalise their problems and who need material aid rather than those with emotional

Juddsy

19074

Pickup By:
16/1/2013

072021

Please remember to issue

this item at the Self service

stations.

Contact us:

Email: Library@bucks.ac.uk

Tel: 01494 605107

Judd

19074

Pickup By:
10/01/2013

072021

Please remember to
issue

this item at the Self
Service

stations.

Contact us:

Email: Library@bucks.ac.
uk

Tel: 01494 605107

Hannah Judd

problems. Only 41 of the 104 MS patients said they had had any contact with a medical social worker, although all patients had at some time attended a hospital clinic and 94 had been in-patients. Some hospital doctors and general practitioners do not view co-ordination with the social services as part of their responsibility to the patient. The survey and subsequent discussions have indicated that some doctors do not know of services and benefits available to the disabled and when they may advise their patients to apply for them, as the following example illustrates:

One patient aged 65 and unmarried had suffered from multiple sclerosis for many years. She could walk only with difficulty and was unable to go out alone from the house where she lived with her 64 year old sister. Because she had a private income no doctor concerned with her management had ever enquired into her financial needs although, as a result of inflation, she was confronted with financial problems as well as difficulty in making social arrangements. At no point had a social work assessment been requested. The patient was recommended to apply for an attendance allowance and arrangements were made for an occupational therapist to visit her home to provide aids, including a wheelchair. The local branch of the Multiple Sclerosis Society was also informed of her interest although she had not previously known of the Society. Information about holidays was given and the Social Work Department in her home area was notified so that a domicilliary visit could be made.

There is some times confusion over applications which had previously been made only by hospital consultants but now can be made by general practitioners on their patients behalf. The example of the general practitioner who did not know that he could apply for an invalid vehicle for his patient has already been quoted (see section on transport p.23).

Continuity of social work support between hospital and home can be achieved by a direct referral of the patient to the local authority social services by the medical social worker. The patient is then known to the local authority and can be registered as disabled even if no services are needed at that stage. When this does not occur, however, a patient who fails to receive hospital follow-up can become lost to the social services. Fifteen of the 41 patients who saw a medical social worker had never had contact with the local authority social work department. Ten of the 15 were found to be in need of social service support ranging from aids and home helps to information on the attendance allowance and day nurseries.

In the present survey the patients were asked if they knew by whom they had been referred to their local social work department. Referrals were found to have come from a variety of sources and in particular district nurses may play an important role in recognising their patients needs and obtaining social work help for them. However, 54 per cent of those known to their local authority had made a direct approach themselves or through a relative and it would seem that under the present arrangements unless patients are prepared to do this, or the local authorities conduct house to house surveys, there is no guarantee that the needs of the disabled living at home will be known. The changes which we recommend would help to overcome this problem (see following section).

Even when a patient is known to a local social work department some of his needs may go unmet because of failures in communication between different workers. Home helps, occupational therapists and social workers all come under the administration of the local authority social work department yet it is possible for a patient to receive help from one of them without a referal to the others where this is appropriate. This occurs most often when a disabled patient expresses a need for an aid. Such a request is usually followed up by an occupational therapist who is able to arrange for the provision of an appliance but who may not be aware of other problems, for example emotional or financial difficulties experienced by the patient. Conversely, social workers who lack a wide knowledge of the aids available to the disabled may fail to seek the advice of the occupational therapist when the provision of an aid may save a patient much frustration and give him more independence. Ten of the 24 patients who were found to be needing aids at the time of the survey had had contact with their local social work department via social workers or home helps but had not been referred to occupational therapists.

Failure of communication between workers and patients about the formers specific roles also caused confusion among patients. Some patients did not know whether the person who visited them from their local authority social work department was a social worker or an occupational therapist and this had to be deduced by the interviewer according to the nature of the help offered to the patient. Patients were also uncertain about the areas of responsibility of the different workers and therefore did not know which problems it was appropriate to discuss with them. Only occasionally did the patients know the names of the workers who had visited them. More care by the workers in explaining the purpose of their visit to the patient, and greater use of professional visiting cards would therefore seem to be justified.

Conclusions and recommendation

There is evidence of many deficiencies in the services which multiple sclerosis sufferers in the West of Scotland are receiving. Few were employed and yet they were not getting full support from the statutory employment services available to them. Social work support was also deficient, for example, many patients who were eligible for the attendance allowance were not receiving it. There was evidence of inadequate liaison between medical and social work teams in the community and hospital and other supporting services, and part of this problem was because those who were least disabled were being followed up more closely by hospital doctors.

We should, however, draw attention to the patchiness of these deficiencies as many patients were receiving some form of help. The overall picture suggested that there was much luck in whether a patient's problems were noticed and that although services were usually available doctors and social workers did not always know about them or when patients were eligible to receive them. The number of MS sufferers in the community is about one in 1200 people, so that any one general practitioner will have only 1 – 3 patients with this disease (McAlpine, Lumsden and Acheson, 1972). There has been evidence that some area authorities have been reluctant to provide help which they should, by law, have made available. This has been due in part to inadequate registration of disabled people. Sometimes local authority officials may have avoided financial and other responsibilities because not sufficient pressure was put upon them. This may have been because the supporting workers dealt with so few patients with MS or similar problems that they were not adequately aware that more should have been done. We suggest that the problem is to a great extent organisational.

At any one time the patients may be visiting or be visited by one or more workers in the social and medical fields including district nurse, LASW, occupational therapist, DRO, etc. In addition the patient may attend hospital and be associated with hospital workers in the same fields. As the diagram (Fig. 13) indicates, at present these people may to a great extent act independently, co-ordination is haphazard and the duplications and deficiences we have described then occur. The help for these patients has been so dissipated that not enough expertise has been developed by the supporting workers.

We suggest that these services should be co-ordinated by the establishment of regular assessment clinics. Registration as a disabled person would mean

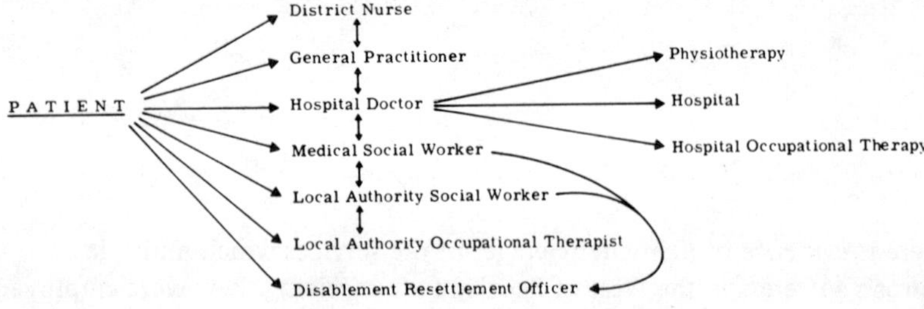

Fig. 13 Diagram of present support services (1976) and their inter-relationships for the physically disabled.

registration at a clinic and hence there would be less risk of loss to follow-up. The clinic would be sited at either a local hospital, rehabilitation centre or health centre depending upon the needs and facilities of the area. It would provide regular assessment and support by being staffed by a doctor, social worker, disablement resettlement officer, occupational therapist and physiotherapist, and the team could hold regular conferences and refer to the hospital doctor and/or general practitioner as necessary (Fig. 14).

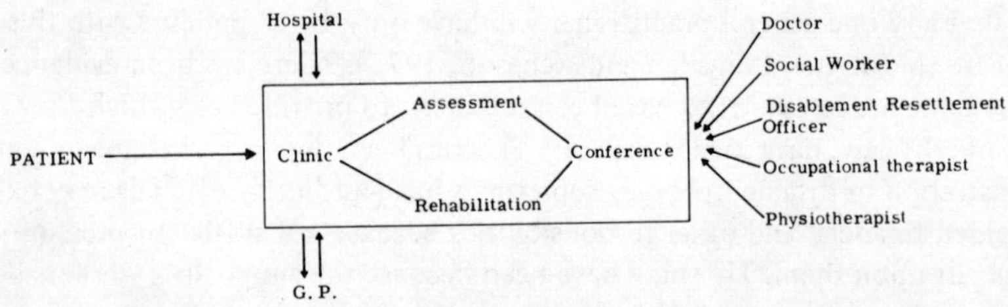

Fig. 14 Rearrangement of support services for the disabled recommended in the Tunbridge report. The major recommendation is the setting up of rehabilitation clinics for assessment of patients.

The concept is not a new one. The Report on Rehabilitation (1972) chaired by Sir Ronald Tunbridge considered:

> In order to foster full communications between the rehabilitation agencies the hospital authorities should set up assessment clinics to cover all hospitals and local authorities within specified areas. . . . The clinic should provide the common basis for all services.

Both the 'Tunbridge' report and the Report on medical rehabilitation in Scotland (chaired by Professor Mair, 1972) pointed out some of the major advantages:

The assessment clinic would

1. be a focal point for rehabilitation services inside and outside the hospital,
2. produce assessment reports,
3. act as a safeguard against patients becoming 'lost' and failing to obtain rehabilitation services,
4. provide training and research opportunity in rehabilitation.

Objections may be raised against reorganisation. Cost might be considered an immediate problem but a reduction in the present duplication of services would be one area of major saving. General practitioners might also feel that this should be part of their service. We would endorse this and suggest that the medical staffing should be by general practitioners who would then develop local expertise for the management of particular diseases. The patchy support by hospital consultants and other medical staff which we have observed would be prevented and their services only called upon for expert opinions or for referal for consideration for inpatient management. Although we argue the need for assessment clinics for sufferers from multiple sclerosis they may also be of value for patients with other chronic diseases who require similar support.

References

Allison, R.S. (1963) Some neurological aspects of medical geography *Proc. Roy. Soc. Med.*, **56**, 71–76

Behan, P.O. and Johnson, R.H. (1975) Autoimmune diseases of the nervous system. *Practitioner,* **214**, 522–532

Bradley, W.G. and Whitty, C.W.M. (1968) Acute optic neuritis : prognosis for development of multiple sclerosis *J. Neurol. Neurosurg. Psychiat.* **31**, 10–18.

Brain, Lord (1962) *Diseases of the Nervous System,* 6th edition, London Oxford University Press

Brown, J.R. (1969) Recent studies in multiple sclerosis. Inference on rehabilitation and employability *Mayo Clin. Proc.* **44**, 758–765

Buckle, J.R. (1971) Work and housing of impaired persons in Great Britain Part II of *Handicapped and Impaired in Great Britain,* H.M.S.O. (London)

Cartlidge, N.E.F. (1972) Autonomic function in multiple sclerosis. *Brain,* **95**, 661–664

Cottrell, S.S. and Kinnier Wilson, S.A. (1927) The affective symptomatology of disseminated sclerosis *J. Neurol. Psychopath.,* **7**, 1.

Davison, A.N., Humphrey, J.H., Liversedge, A.L., McDonald, W.I. and Porterfield, J.S. (Eds.) (1975) *Multiple Sclerosis Research,* H.M.S.O. (London)

Dean, G. (1975) Epidemiology: what is new and what remains to be done *Multiple Sclerosis Research* (Ed. Davison, A.N., Humphrey, J.H., Liversedge, A.L., McDonald, W.I., Porterfield, J.S.), H.M.S.O. (London)

Editorial, (1972) Benign forms of multiple sclerosis *Brit. Med. J.,* **i**, 392

Forder, A., Reti, T., Silver, J.R. (1969) Communication in the health service: a case study of the rehabilitation of paraplegic patients *Social and Economic Administration* **3**, 1, 3–16

Fryers, T., Banning, B. and Newton, P. (1974) *The Chronic Sick and Handicapped in Salford.* 2 part survey, University of Manchester Department of Community Medicine, Salford Department of Social services, private circulation

Goldsmith, S. (1967) *Designing for the Disabled* Royal Institute of British Architects, London, 207 pp.

Greengross, W. (1976) *Entitled to love. The Sexual and Emotional Needs of the Handicapped.* Malaby Press in association with the National Fund for Research into Crippling Diseases, 128 pp.

Gregory, E. (1973) Implementing the chronically sick and disabled persons act. *Social Work Today,* 4, 11, 351

Harris, A.I. (1971) Handicapped and impaired in Great Britain Part I Office of Population Censuses and Surveys. H.M.S.O. (London)

Johnson, R.H. and Johnson, G.S. (1972) Differences in opportunities for the disabled in England and Scotland: a survey of paraplegics in Scotland *Brit. Med. J.,* **1**, 779–782

Johnson G.S. and Johnson, R.H. (1973) Paraplegics in Scotland: a survey of employment and facilities *Br. J. Social Wk.,* **3** (1) 19–38

Johnson G.S. and Johnson R.H. (1977) Social Services support for multiple sclerosis patients in the West of Scotland, *Lancet,* **1**, 31–34

Johnson, R.H. and McLellan, D.L. (1972) Multiple Sclerosis: a Review *The Practitioner,* **209**, 183–190

Kurtzke, J.F., Beebe, G.W., Nagler, B., Nefzger, M.D., Auth, T.L. and Kurland, L.T. (1970) Studies on the natural history of multiple sclerosis, Section 5, long term survival in young men *Archs. Neurol.,* **22**, 215–225

Lynes, T. (1972) Wheelchair power. *New Society,* 10th August, p.290

McAlpine, D. (1973) Multiple Sclerosis: a review *Brit. Med. J.,* **2**, 292–295

McAlpine, D., Lumsden, C.E. and Acheson, E.D. (1972) *Multiple Sclerosis: a Reappraisal* 2nd edn. Edinburgh: Livingstone.

McCallum, J. (1973) The social consequences of multiple sclerosis Report to the National Multiple Sclerosis Society of New Zealand Inc. on a survey carried out in 1971–72.

McCallum, J. (1973) The social consequences of multiple sclerosis Report to the National Multiple Sclerosis Society of New Zealand Inc.

Panelius, M. (1969) Studies on epidemiological, clinical and etiological aspects of multiple sclerosis, *Acta. Neurol. Scand.,* Suppl. **39**, 1–82.

Percy, A.K., Nobrega, F.T., Okazaki, H., Glattre, E. and Kurland, L.T. (1971) Multiple sclerosis in Rochester, Minnesota *Archs. Neurol.* **25**, 105–111

Report (1972) Medical Rehabilitation: the pattern for the future Report of a sub-committee of the standing medical advisory committee (chairman Mair, A.), Scottish Home and Health Department, H.M.S.O. (Edinburgh)

Report (1975) Multiple Sclerosis No. 52 in a series of papers on current health problems, Office of Health Economics, London

Report (1972) Rehabilitation, Report of a sub-committee of the standing medical advisory committee (chairman: Tunbridge, Sir Ronald), Department of Health and Social Security, H.M.S.O. (London)

Report (1974) Report and recommendations of the National Advisory Commission on multiple sclerosis, vols. 1 and 2 U.S. Department of Health, Education and Welfare, Public Health Service, National Institutes of Health, DHEW Publication No. (NIH) 74–534

Report (1975) *The Census Indicators of Urban Poverty* Department of Environment and Home Office Urban Deprivation Unit

Report (1973) *The Implementation of the Chronically Sick and Disabled Persons Act 1970* Social Policy Research Unit report published by the National Fund for Crippling Diseases, Horsham, Sussex.

Report (1975) *The Missing Million. Have they been found?* A report on the conference organised on progress in searching out people who are eligible for services under the Chronically Sick and Disabled Persons Act 1970 National Fund for Research into Crippling Diseases, Horsham, Sussex.

Stevens, B.C. (1974) A pilot enquiry on the social and psychological needs of patients disabled by multiple sclerosis and other neurological diseases *Rehabilitation* No. 90 41–49 *(Journal of the British Council for Rehabilitation of the Disabled)*

Surridge, D. (1969) An investigation into some psychiatric aspects of multiple sclerosis *British J. Psychiat.,* **115**, 749–764.

Walton, J.N. (1977) *Brain's Diseases of the Nervous System,* 8th edn. London: Oxford University Press.